What People Are Saying

"The person to call for guided travel to Utah's National Parks"

- *DEPARTURES* **Magazine**

"One of the Top Trainers in the Industry"

- **The Sports Club/LA**, Washington, D.C. (now Equinox)

"If you ever need an amazing tour guide for
Utah, reach out to Melanie Webb."

- **Vic Gundotra**, V.P. of Engineering, Google

"I've known Melanie for more than a decade and her knowledge
of fitness combined with her passion for the outdoors makes her
an excellent facilitator for outdoor-based fitness programs."

- **Pete McCall**, Fitness Author and Instructor at Mesa College

"Melanie Webb and her program have coached and guided me
every step of the way as I launch my new fitness adventure
service. As a business owner and a mom, my time is limited
and *Adventures in Mother Nature's Gym* has provided a unique,
cutting edge forum to allow me to learn at my own pace."

- **Chris Kirchoff**, MA, ACSM HI-FI and Owner, Kirchoff Fitness

"What Melanie Webb offers in her *Adventures in Mother Nature's Gym* is a program that can help reconnect our patients and clients to an aspect of their being that is undernourished and therefore contributing to their depleted state. Melanie makes being in the outdoors fun, playful, and yet pragmatic."
- **Karen Koffler**, M.D., Medical Director of the Osher Integrative Medical Center at the University of Miami, Miami, Florida

"Melanie Webb introduced me to wilderness with hiking trips to Zion National Park and Machu Picchu, Peru. Now, when I'm out of sync with Mother Nature, I'm out of sync with everything."
- **Amie Kane-Lee**, Muscle Activation Technique Specialist and Owner, Peak Performance

"Running my small business from the road isn't easy, and comes with a lot of stress. Attending a Sol Fitness Adventure in Utah was just what I needed to unwind and re-connect with nature. The techniques I learned there improved the fitness of both my body & mind."
- **Matthew Karsten**, The Expert Vagabond

"This course is well thought out and challenges the reader's critical thinking skills by empowering them to put theory into action. Melanie's qualifications alone make the book stand out as a credible resource."

- **Sarah Anisman**, M.S. Kinesiology and Sport Psychology, Owner of Yoga Lab Mammoth

"What can you get out of it? This type of 'workout' is at a minimum, a reward for – or culmination of – all of the other routine workouts that you have done—'applied conditioning' if you will, where you can see the benefits of your efforts under unique conditions."

- **Jeff Tassey**, Tassey and Associates

"The philosophies and pragmatic instruction in this book certainly comport with the standard of care for musculoskeletal health. As a member of the Board of Counselors at the American Academy of Orthopaedic Surgery, I can strongly state that if the world followed the precepts espoused in this book, fewer people would require the skills that I can offer in clinic or in the operating room."

- **Paul Winterton** M.D., Board of Counselors, American Academy of Orthopaedic Surgeons

Adventures in

MOTHER NATURE'S GYM

The Ultimate Guide to
Planning & Leading Your Own
Outdoor Fitness Retreats

MELANIE WEBB
2019

ALSO BY MELANIE WEBB

Adventures in MOTHER NATURE'S GYM The Business Workbook: The

Ultimate Guide to Monetizing Your Own Outdoor Fitness Retreats

Sol Guide: Online Training for Your Next Outdoor Fitness Trip

Mother Nature's Gym

Confessions of a Tour Guide

Slot Canyon Body Slam

Adventures in

MOTHER NATURE'S GYM

The Ultimate Guide to
Planning & Leading Your Own
Outdoor Fitness Retreats

MELANIE WEBB

Owner of Sol Fitness Adventures and ACE-Certified Personal Trainer

Published by Sol Fitness Adventures, dba WebbWell
WebbWell.com

ISBN 9781791962548

The exercise program and other information contained in this book should not be followed without first consulting your health care professional and the laws of your State relating to Certified Personal Trainers, mind/body instructors and Outfitters and Guides.

To the many 'clients' and 'guests,' both indoors and out, who have entrusted

me with their health and safety, friendship and love, and without

whom so many grand adventures would not have been possible.

Contents

"Who needs wilderness?

Civilization needs wilderness!"

- EDWARD ABBEY, from *Freedom and Wilderness, Wilderness and Freedom*

FOREWORD

by **Karen Koffler, M.D.**, *Medical Director of the Osher Integrative*

Medical Center at the University of Miami, Miami, Florida

As an Integrative and Functional medicine physician, I often see people who have chronic health issues that are eroding their quality of life. When I delve into their lifestyle, I hear a recurrent theme of over-commitment, lack of attention to their own personal needs, and a real disengagement from their natural bio-rhythms. Coupled with the growing anxiety and addiction I see related to being connected to the news and digital devices—I worry about the tsunami of worsening health in the United States of America.

Living on an island, I often use the beach as a therapeutic tool. "Spend twenty minutes at the ocean" is a common recommendation for many of my patients as a way for them to get sunlight and hence vitamin D, negative ions from the waves, and the peace that comes from the open vista, muted sounds, salt air, and the rocking movement of the water. For those who take me up on it, it is often their best medicine.

To handle modern day stress and its inevitable toll on our psyche and soma, those of us in healthcare will need to become more creative in how we help those entrusted to us not just survive, but thrive. A pill is not going to treat the vague and pervasive disease that is only increasing in our society and is a major contributor to the epidemics of obesity, heart disease, diabetes, dementia, depression, anxiety, and more.

What Melanie Webb offers in her series *Adventures in Mother Nature's Gym* is a program that will help reconnect our patients and clients to an aspect of their being that is undernourished and therefore contributing to their depleted state. Melanie makes being in the outdoors fun, playful, and yet pragmatic. It is obvious in this well-thought out manual, and I can personally attest to the value of this approach, having gone on retreat with Melanie in Utah with my own children (then ages 10 and 11). Six years later, we still reflect on that experience that allowed us to explore the wilderness, connect us to a place, and have a fun adventure while learning about the Colorado Plateau and Southern Utah. As a testament to its lasting effects, we continue to create vacations that incorporate that same experience. And after each one, we feel more peaceful and yet energized than any other kind of travel.

INTRODUCTION

I'm excited to share what I've gathered during my 20-year career working in fitness and the outdoors.

As a Certified Personal Trainer with the American Council on Exercise (ACE), I'm also a big fan of Eastern modalities including qigong, yoga, and a variety of meditation and stress reduction techniques. As a former wildlife biologist I also draw from activities designed to enhance observation skills and foster a curiosity of the natural world. The result is a compilation of collective teachings and ideas combined and organized into the method that I use to guide customized outdoor fitness retreats through my small company Sol Fitness Adventures. To keep things simple for this course I'll call my practice Sol Guide Method..

During the last 13 years of running outdoor fitness retreats I have often felt like a maverick. My own clients initially asked me to take them on fitness retreats that combined traditional exercise methods with different forms of outdoor adventures, like hiking and biking. While it was right in my wheelhouse I couldn't find anyone else who was doing this hybrid type of work at a highly customized level of expertise. The closest alternative for my clients was a spa trip—and they'd already 'been there, done that.' It meant that there was a lot of trial and error - especially in finding the right markets to tap into as I tried to grow my business beyond my existing client base. I spent a few years moonlighting as a hiking, canyoneering, and cycling guide for other adventure travel companies while I bootstrapped my own fledgling business, which, while it was rewarding in many ways, also felt like a tremendous sacrifice of time and money.

I watched and waited for the day that an understanding of the importance of nature to our health and wellbeing would become mainstream. I reached out to and met with thought leaders who inspired me and continued to refine my method with each new trip. Eventually I reached a point where I realized that I'd learned a great deal, and that maybe it was time for me to stop waiting for others to do the work and to take the leap of confidence to start the conversation with the fitness industry myself.

Sandy Webster, Editor of *IDEA Fitness Journal*, accepted my pitch to contribute an article, and *Mother Nature's Gym* was published in the May 2014 issue. I heard from several fitness trainers and group exercise instructors who wanted to start leading their own fitness retreats. I was thrilled and consulted with them to set up their own practice.

Helping those trainers plan and execute their own international fitness adventures and treks inspired me, and convinced me that there were more people out there who could use this information.

Fitness retreats bridge the gap between indoor fitness workouts and outdoor active adventures and are a valuable tool to help people rediscover and nurture their own relationship to the body and the planet in the 21st Century. I don't claim any exclusive ownership over the concepts presented here. I don't feel that there's one right way to approach fitness or one method to train every client who crosses my path. What I do know is that having a natural curiosity has added to my 'bag of training tricks' and kept my passion for this field burning bright.

What You Will Learn

Adventures in MOTHER NATURE'S GYM will give you tools to help your clients reclaim that instinctive, wild, and very necessary part of the human experience—adventure! Like most great books, it won't take anything away from your existing expertise and knowledge base, but it certainly will add to it. With the skills you learn here you'll expand on your existing mind/body practice and connect with the outdoors in new and exciting ways. As a result you'll attract a continuous flow of clients who seek opportunities to transform not only the shape of their body, but also the very fabric of their way of life.

Everyone comes to the fitness industry with different passions, backgrounds, and skills. How you integrate the methods presented in this course into your existing business model will vary. Regardless of whether you specialize in private fitness, group recreation, or a clinical setting, *Adventures in MOTHER NATURE'S GYM* contains a set of tools that everyone can learn and apply to their own specialty.

You'll learn the latest scientific research of how and why being outdoors benefits the human body and mind. You'll review the basic principles of designing an exercise program – such as sport specific warm-ups and cool downs – and learn how to combine them with real outdoor adventures like hiking, cycling, and stand up paddling to create your own outdoor fitness retreats. An essential component of the course is the exercise library, the 'Body-Weight Exercise Arsenal.' Found in Part Six, the library includes photos and verbal cues to over 40 full-body movements that don't require equipment and can be performed in any outdoor setting. Bonus material includes exclusive access to the accompanying instructional video library found on the Sol Fitness Adventures website at http://solfitnessadventures.com/mother-natures-gym-exercise-arsenal/

IMPORTANT!

Adventures in MOTHER NATURE'S GYM teaches you how to:

1. Design, plan and lead your own outdoor fitness retreats using Sol Guide Method
2. Combine fitness program design with guided outdoor excursions
3. Harness the inherent health and wellness benefits of nature
4. Develop the skill-sets of an outdoor fitness guide
5. Enhance your own connection to Mother Nature and the outdoors

Who Can Benefit from Reading *Adventures in MOTHER NATURE'S GYM*?

Fitness trainers and mind-body instructors can come from many backgrounds and disciplines, and that variety is what makes the industry so powerful. The Sol Guide Method introduced in *Adventures in MOTHER NATURE'S GYM* integrates with many different specialties and disciplines and improves the overall fitness offerings available to clients. Of course, the variety of backgrounds can also create some challenges. I share this training method under the assumption that you already possess a baseline level of knowledge and proficiency in your area of expertise and in safely implementing fitness programs.

Disciplines that compliment this method include:

1. Certified Personal Trainers and Group Fitness Instructors
2. Mind-body instructors including yoga and Pilates teachers
3. Muscle Activation Therapists (MAT)
4. Wellness and Nutrition Coaches

5. Martial arts instructors including Brazilian Capoeira, Jiu Jitsu, Thai Chi and Qi Gong
6. Adventure travel guides and recreation management experts
7. Counselors, therapists and physicians

In other words, if you're an existing member of the community of people around the world who are striving to help people live healthier lives, this course is for you!

First Aid

I assume that you already possess a working knowledge of the human body, healthy movement, and your own specialty form of exercise instruction. I'll build off of that specialized knowledge and teach you the conceptual information and practical skills you need to be able to take your specialty and combine it with outdoor adventures.

If you are currently instructing any form of fitness or mind/body program you should already have a current Basic First Aid/CPR certification. While this is sufficient for indoor disciplines, to safely guide paying clients in the outdoors ultimately requires more in-depth first aid training. The minimum level of acceptable first aid training recommended for leading a fitness retreat is Wilderness First Aid (WFA). Later in the course you will learn about different levels of first aid certification in detail, so you'll be able to determine which additional training may be right for you.

Why *Adventures in MOTHER NATURE'S GYM?*

As I watch the developed world become more digitized—yet at the same time stricken with mental illness and preventable disease states—I worry that we're losing something, an energy that has existed since man stood on two feet and walked upright. At the same time, I hear science and mainstream culture engaging in the conversation that a connection to the outdoors is an important aspect of being human. Is that what we've lost—the wild part of human nature, the sense that life is one big *adventure?*

Think about it: as a fitness industry we encourage people to come into buildings and stand on electric machinery to move. It appears as if most people aren't moving at all unless they schedule that time to 'exercise.' And yet, how many years did man exist on the planet without gyms and yoga studios?

Fitness Meets Adventure

If what I propose sounds a little disruptive to the institutionalized fabric of fitness in the 'civilized' world, then good! Let's shake things up a little and return to our own wild and instinctive connection to this planet we call home. Bring your existing certifications and knowledge to the table, learn a few new things here, and then show the rest of us what you can create that helps your community (and the world) live a more integrated and adventurous life!

Key Terms

Adventure – An unusual and exciting, sometimes-hazardous experience or activity calling for enterprise and enthusiasm.

Disruptive – Changing the traditional way that an industry operates, especially in a new and effective way.[1]

Adventure Travel – A trip that has a mix of culture, nature and activity, which can range from very serene to very extreme.[2]

Will this transform the way you train or run your practice now? I suspect it probably will – for the better. Am I asking you to abandon your indoor practice and replace it with the untamed wilderness? No way! But I do think that as you complete this course you will begin to think of additional ways to add a sense of adventure that compliments your existing practice.

This course will blow the walls and the roof off of what your current scope of practice allows – and doesn't allow – you to do with your clients. What new doors will this course open for you? For one, the entire world will become your gym. You will no longer be limited to earning money indoors as you count down the hours and the number of reps until your last client goes home at the end of the day so that you can go outside for that liberating run or bike ride. *Adventures in MOTHER NATURE'S GYM* will breathe new life into a setting that can become stale and redundant; the never-ending hamster wheel of showing up to the studio at 6am and being limited to getting paid by the hour. Learn the material in this course well and you will be able to expand your office to include the great outdoors and diversify the way you earn money.

Don't Forget the Accompaniment Workbook

Adventures in MOTHER NATURE'S GYM: The Business Workbook will walk you step by step through packaging and selling your own customized outdoor fitness retreat. With the toolkit you'll receive in The Business Workbook, you'll be prepared to break free from the hourly confines of the indoor gyms and studios and earn even more money doing what you love – sharing your passion for the active lifestyle with others.

The Business Workbook teaches you how to:

1. Build fitness retreats into an existing mind/body business practice
2. Mitigate risks and navigate the legalities of operating in the outdoors
3. Research and implement business and liability insurance requirements
4. Create gear lists, safety talks, and client intake forms
5. Brand, market, and sell a retreat tailored to your community

After you complete both books you will be prepared to plan and guide your own outdoor fitness retreat. You can start small with a local Saturday afternoon event and see how it goes. If it's a big success and you enjoyed the process, you can add one retreat each quarter, or try planning a local adventure each month.

My Story

I wasn't trying to disrupt the fitness or outdoor industries when I stumbled onto this work back in 2007. I was busy building my clientele as a personal trainer. I'd been certified through ACE (American Council on Exercise) for seven years and was an Advantage Trainer through NASM (National Academy of Sports Medicine). Prior to that, when I graduated from college in Utah and decided not to go to physical therapy school, I fell back on all the undergrad research I did in school and went to work as a Wildlife Biologist for the Utah Division of Wildlife Resources. I enjoyed working to save endangered species and loved exploring remote parts of the state. A scientist at heart, the research and writing came easy to me.

But I wasn't fulfilled working in wildlife. I'd studied the human body, been an athlete my entire life, and dreamed of helping people be healthy. I took my test to become a personal trainer and went to work a few nights a week at a private training studio. Fitness trainers weren't in hot demand at the time. I kept at it part-time while my biology career progressed and I was offered a job as an Environmental Consultant in Washington, D.C. – working for the Feds!

I'd never wanted to move back east, but I'm also not one to turn down an opportunity. I accepted the offer and took a sabbatical from fitness training. I was a complete fish out of water. Instead of working with endangered species I was navigating bureaucracy, pushing papers and sitting in a cubicle all day! Though I enjoyed my new city and making the big bucks I knew the life behind a desk was not for me.

I decided to recommit to fitness and applied to graduate programs in exercise science. My consulting contract fulfilled, I said goodbye to my five-year wildlife career and dove into an advanced exercise science degree at The George Washington University. By that time I'd been out of school for six years. It felt strange not to work. I started training again at the Sports Club/LA (now Equinox) and before I knew it I was booked solid. I was stoked to be training again and spent the next six years doing it, full time.

It was during a training session in 2007 that a client said to me, "Melanie, I want to take an active vacation to Deer Valley with my niece, and I want you to lead it." She'd cycled around the world with the best-known travel companies and been to all the best spas. She wanted to apply the training we'd been doing in the gym to real life and spend time training at high altitude to prepare for her ski season.

With her input I planned a multi-sport four-day trip to my home state of Utah. It turned out that another client owned a boutique hotel at Deer Valley, so I worked out a deal with her on rooms. I already knew the best hikes and bike routes in the area, so all I had to do was figure out where to rent the bikes, how we'd get around, and how much all of this was going to cost. I leaned on the experience from my old days as a wildlife biologist, when I used to look at a map, pick a stream, organize my crew, the food and gear, and drive four hours to the middle of a desert to conduct field research.

Our trip to Utah was a big success. Each morning we did a small workout on the deck overlooking the ski resort. Then we'd ride bikes into the Uinta Forest or hike a 12,000 ft mountain. The chef taught us how to make fondue and my clients had a massage every day. She met her goals of challenging herself and spending quality time with her niece before she went off to college.

I had a blast planning and guiding the trip. It felt like I'd recaptured the active outdoor lifestyle I'd had before I moved to the big city. I loved sharing what I knew with others and I enjoyed the change of venue from the city gym. I wasn't trying to create a new career for myself, but when my other clients heard about the trip they wanted their own special Utah adventure too! It slowly started to snowball.

Fast forward to today and here I am, sharing what I've gathered along my journey. I've included a few personal stories from my own experiences that I hope share nuggets of hard-earned wisdom.

Tag your adventures on social media with #MotherNaturesGym to spark ideas and inspire the rest of us!

HOW TO USE THIS BOOK

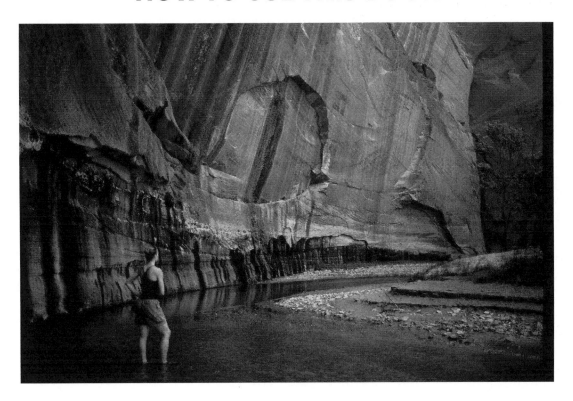

The theories I share in this book are the heart of what I call Sol Guide Method and work best when paired with my book *Adventures in MOTHER NATURE'S GYM: The Business Workbook, The Ultimate Guide to Monetizing Your Own Outdoor Fitness Retreats*, which contains content and instruction related to monetizing and insuring an outdoor fitness retreat. Throughout this book you'll encounter a variety of practice quizzes that are designed to enhance the learning and retention of the concepts presented in each chapter. You won't be graded so have fun with these—know that they provide the opportunity for you to review and interact with key topics that will help you succeed. Part Six contains the Body-Weight Exercise Arsenal, my favorite exercises to use on Sol Fitness Adventures. You will also receive exclusive complimentary access to the instructional video library found on my website at http://solfitnessadventures.com/mother-natures-gym-exercise-arsenal/

Please, reach out and share how you're using these tools to improve the lives of your own community and clients. Email me at info@solfitnessadventures.com and tag your adventures using #mothernaturesgym on social media. Your successes and adventures will inspire and give the rest of us encouragement as we work to improve the health and well-being of our clients, our communities, and our planet.

Melanie Webb

TYPES OF LEARNING EXERCISES

Both this book and *Mother Nature's Gym: The Business Manual* contain seven types of learning exercises: matching, multiple choice, fill in the blank, true or false, crossword puzzles, word searches, and journal entries. Instructions for each type of exercise are explained below.

Matching
Matching exercises ask you to match the terms listed in one column or above each sentence with the corresponding descriptive phrase. Each term will be used only once.

Multiple Choice
This exercise presents a statement or question followed by answers lettered 'a' through 'd' presenting various options. Select the letter that corresponds to the correct answer.

Fill In The Blank
This exercise asks you to write in the missing word or words in a statement using the list of words or phrases provided. There are more words listed than there are blank spaces.

True or False
A statement is presented, and you are asked to determine whether the statement is true or false.

Crossword Puzzles
The crossword puzzles are made up of words taken from key concepts throughout the chapter that preceded it and are made of words spelled both vertically and horizontally.

Word Searches
The word searches contain complete words amidst a series of randomly generated letters. The words are selected from important concepts within the chapter in which it is located. Try looking at the word search as a whole and see what words pop out at you.

Journal Entries

Journal entries guide you through a creative process of formulating your own retreat, so that by the time you finish reading, you are ready to put a plan into action. Use the small amount of space provided to take notes that will spur your memory. You may wish to answer the thought questions more in depth by recording your answers in a separate notebook or on a computer.

CHECKING YOUR ANSWERS

Once you've completed the quizzes in each chapter, check your answers against the Answer Key included at the end of this workbook. You won't be graded, but if you answer a question incorrectly it's a good idea to go back and re-read sections as a review. The review process will help create a checklist of important steps to complete as you package and prepare to sell a retreat to paying clients.

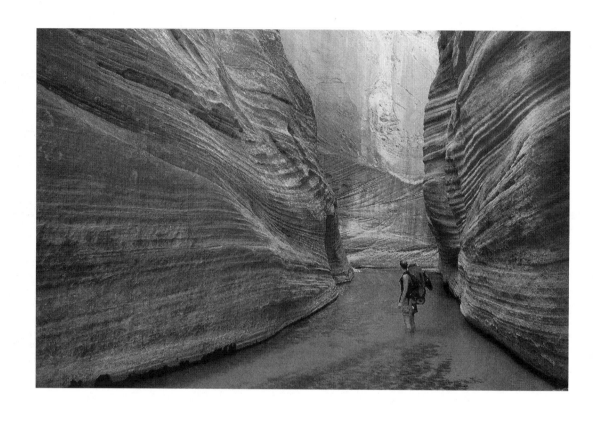

PART ONE
THE NEED FOR CREATIVE FITNESS SOLUTIONS

"We are not defined by our many scars, but by

what we do after the wounds close."

– MICAH FINK, HEROES AND HORSES

The world is full of 'quick and easy' ways to improve health and 'lose the weight fast.' You hear them every day on the radio and see them in sponsored internet ads: "Take this pill made from the rare, exotic narwhalberry." Or, "Use the Ab Annihilator for three minutes a day and you can have a six pack by Wednesday."

We know that get-healthy-quick schemes aren't the answer. True health and well-being requires more than simply losing the weight, but many people don't know what it feels like to be truly healthy. So what are the obstacles standing in the way of us living our most healthy, vibrant lives? In this chapter I'll examine four of the major hurdles to wellness, including:

- sedentary lifestyle and obesity
- mental health disorders
- digital distraction
- nature deficit disorder

I'll cover each in depth and reveal how the Sol Guide Method works to combat these threats to our well-being.

Sedentary Lifestyle and Obesity

You know from the news that people and communities face a wide array of health and wellness obstacles. Many of the traditional solutions—healthy diet, exercise, and stress reduction—have not been successful with the population as a whole.

One of the biggest threats to the health of the American people is a sedentary lifestyle. What do I mean by sedentary lifestyle? You may have heard of the term "couch potato" to describe someone who sits on the couch watching TV and eats junk food all day. Nowadays even working professionals sitting in the office day after day may fall into sedentary habits. Someone who is said to lead a sedentary life has little and irregular physical activity. Many people who lead a sedentary lifestyle may also fall into the category of being obese.

The terms obesity and overweight refer to ranges of weight generally considered to be greater than that considered healthy for any given height and which are directly correlated to a variety of illnesses, including:

- diabetes
- hypertension
- stroke
- obesity

Diabetes – A disorder of carbohydrate metabolism characterized by inadequate production or utilization of insulin and resulting in excessive amounts of glucose in the blood and urine.

Hypertension – Elevation of the blood pressure, especially the diastolic pressure.

Stroke – Sudden, focal interruption of cerebral blood flow that causes neurologic deficit. Symptoms and signs: occur suddenly, numbness, weakness or paralysis of contralateral limbs and face, confusion, visual disturbances, dizziness, loss of balance, headache.[3]

Obesity – Body weight in excess of biological needs; excessive fatness. Moderate obesity is 20 or 30% - 100% above ideal body weight.[4]

Table 1. Classification based on measures of diastolic and systolic blood pressure.

CLASSIFICATION	BP (MMHG)
Normal	< 120/80
Prehypertension	120 – 139 / 80 – 89
Stage 1	140 – 159 (systolic) or 90 – 99 (diastolic)
Stage 2	> 160 (systolic)

The Center for Disease Control and Prevention (CDC) reported that 4 in 10 adults age 20 and over were obese in 2015-2016, compared with 3 in 10 in 2001 – 2002.[5] A separate CDC report cited the following population statistics for the years 2013-2014:

- 37.9% of adults aged 20 and over were obese
- 70.7% adults ages 20 and over were overweight and obese.
- 20.6% adolescents ages 12-19 years were obese
- 17.4% of children ages 6-11 years were obese
- 9.4% of children ages 2-5 were obese[6]

Mental Health Disorders

While the obesity epidemic threatens populations both young and old, there is also an alarming increase in the diagnosis of mental health disorders. Most of us have friends and/or family members who suffer from something on this list, if not ourselves at some point in our lives. Given the prevalence of these disorders, you are bound to have clients who are also afflicted and who need your empathy and understanding. Good for them for including exercise in their self-care plan! While we won't go into mental illness in great depth, it's important to be familiar with some of the more common diagnoses. The Diagnostic and Statistical Manual of Mental Disorders[7] (DSM-V) defines the following categories and related disorders:

- Anxiety disorders – Include post-traumatic stress disorder (PTSD), generalized anxiety disorder and phobias
- Depression – Includes unipolar depression and bipolar depression
- Eating disorders – Includes anorexia nervosa, binge eating disorder, and bulimia nervosa
- Personality disorders – Includes antisocial personality disorder, avoidant personality disorder, and borderline personality disorder

IMPORTANT!

- The National Comorbidity Study Replication (NCS-R) data indicated that among U.S. adults aged 18 or older the prevalence of any anxiety disorder during the past year was 19%,[8] with an estimated 31.1% experiencing any anxiety disorder at some point in their lifetime.[9]
- Data gathered from the World Economic Forum in 2010 reported that mental disorders were the largest cost driver at $2.5 trillion in global costs, greater than the costs of diabetes, respiratory disorders, and cancer combined.[10]
- The National Health and Nutrition Examination Survey, 2009 – 2012, reported 7.6% of Americans aged 12 and over had depressive symptoms within the past two weeks.[11]

Post-traumatic stress disorder (PTSD) – Development of characteristic symptoms following exposure to one or more traumatic events. The clinical presentation includes fear-based experiencing, emotional and behavioral symptoms among other symptom patterns. The traumatic event can be experienced in various ways. Individuals with PTSD may be quick tempered and may engage in aggressive verbal and/or physical behavior with little or no provocation. May engage in recklessness or self-injurious or suicidal behavior.

Generalized Anxiety Disorder (GAD) – Excessive anxiety and worry, occurring more days than not for at least six months, about a number of events or activities. Difficulty controlling the worry. Associated with three or more of the following:

- Restlessness
- Easily fatigued
- Difficulty concentrating
- Irritability
- Muscle tension
- Sleep disturbance

Phobias – Individuals with specific phobias are fearful or anxious about or avoidant of circumscribed objects or situations. The fear, anxiety, or avoidance is almost always immediately induced by the phobic situation, various types of:

- Animals
- Natural environments
- Situations
- Social settings
- Crowd settings

Unipolar Depression – Common feature of all depressive disorders is the presence of sad, empty, or irritable mood, accompanied by somatic and cognitive changes that significantly affect the individual's capacity to function. Differences among them are issues of duration, timing, or presumed etiology.

Eating Disorders – Psychological illnesses defined by abnormal eating habits that may involve either insufficient or excessive food intake to the detriment of an individual's physical and mental health.

Addiction – Substance-related disorders encompass 10 separate classes of drugs. All drugs taken in excess have in common the direct activation of the brain reward system, which is involved in the reinforcement of behaviors and the production of memories. They produce such an intense activation of the reward system that normal activities may be neglected. Other excessive behavioral patterns such as gambling, Internet gaming, sex addiction, exercise and shopping addictions are not included in the DSM-V due to insufficient peer reviewed evidence.

Digital Distraction

Have you given any thought to how much time you or your clients spend each day on your smart phones and other digital devices? I'm going to guess that you're the kind of person who has done more than just think about it every now and then. When I wrote the first edition of this course in 2013 digital distraction was a relatively new term used to describe our growing over-dependence on digital devices. Research published in the *IDEA Fitness Journal* in June 2013 showed that overuse of electronic media elevates stress, reduces concentration and productivity and elicits an addiction response in the brain. Author Shirley Archer wrote, "Some think that constant media engagement is one of the most serious threats to humanity."[12]

Now, you might find the 'threat to humanity' assessment to be a bit extreme. Try explaining that to people who visit The Die With Me chat room, the app you can only use when your mobile device has less that 5% battery.[13] Writer Tripp Mickle explained "nomophobia, short for no-mobile-phobia" as the term used to describe the fear people feel when they run out of mobile contact entirely. Mickle went on to report that since 2014 close to 15 papers have been published on nomophobia, with twice as many papers published on phone-related anxieties since 2016.[14]

While I'm lucky not to suffer from nomophobia I can certainly relate to worrying about my cell phone battery staying charged. I take an extra battery pack when I travel or spend extended time in the outdoors – just in case. My friends and clients and I discuss the need to 'unplug' on a regular basis now, and the scientific interest and findings on the impact of technology on our well-being fascinates me.

We can expect to see a continued rise in anxiety disorders as technology occupies more time during our daily lives. Interestingly, exercise is suggested as one of the leading ways to counter too much media exposure and anxiety disorders. You can help your clients unplug more frequently and in meaningful ways as you lead them into playful, fun, engaging outdoor fitness activities.

JOURNAL ENTRY - DIGITAL DISTRACTION

How would you assess the impact of digital devices on your personal health and well-being?

What about your clients, do you think any of them suffer from nomophobia or digital-related anxiety?

Have you ever intentionally unplugged from your devices?

Write down some ways that you can combat digital distraction in yours and your clients' lives.

The following crossword puzzle reviews the negative impact digital distraction can have on overall health.

Crossword

Complete the sentences below by selecting the correct term and writing it in the appropriate box in the crossword puzzle.

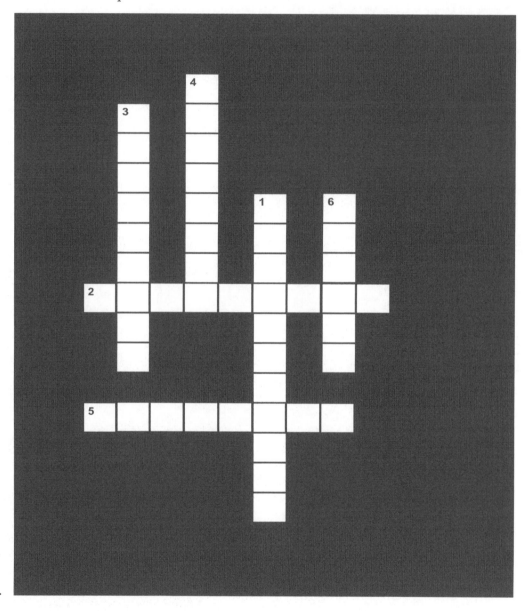

Descriptions

1. The over-dependence on digital devices is called digital _____.

2. Excessive use of digital devices contributes to both a sedentary _____ and anxiety disorders.

3. The continual use of digital devices can elicit an _____ response in the brain.

4. One of the leading ways to counter the negative impact of media exposure is _____.

5. Overuse of electronic media can cause _____ stress.

6. It is a good idea to help your clients _____ frequently and lead them to engaging outdoor activities.

Nature Deficit Disorder

So far in this chapter I've covered three major hurdles to health:

- sedentary lifestyle
- mental health issues
- digital distraction

These hurdles don't typically occur in isolation. Often they are intertwined. People spend too much time on their digital devices, contributing to a sedentary lifestyle and even, possibly, mental health disorders including anxiety and depression. The results are a modern phenomenon that researcher and author Richard Louv has called nature deficit disorder. [15]

Nature deficit disorder is directly connected to our growing over-dependence on technology and sedentary lifestyles. The term includes the wide range of behavioral problems that stem from humans spending less time outdoors, a condition that applies to both children and adults. Now a commonly used term among health practitioners and child development specialists, the effects of the disorder include:

- disengagement from nature
- attention disorders
- depression
- poor performance in school

The implications of nature deficit disorder extend beyond the individual to affect entire societies. Author Tri Robinson said, "One of the main drivers of poverty on the planet is a non-sustainable environment."[16] Raising a generation of children who don't interact with the outdoors will have a negative impact on the world's green energy efforts, environmental and conservation movements, commitment to organic eating, and sustainable farming and growing practices.

Combating Nature Deficit Disorder

In Louv's acclaimed book *Last Child in the Woods*, he makes two suggestions for health care providers: "In the ongoing search for answers to child obesity . . . health care practitioners...should emphasize free outdoor play, especially in natural surroundings, as much as they do organized sports . . ."[17] You have a tremendous opportunity to help people combat nature deficit disorder as you begin leading your own outdoor fitness retreats. Whether you choose to work with children, families, or primarily adults, the act of introducing more people to the outdoor lifestyle will have a far-reaching impact.

Through my work with the outdoor industry I've been privileged to attend two different keynote speeches from one of my personal heroes, Former Secretary of the Department of the Interior Sally Jewell. Secretary Jewell was actively involved in the nature deficit conversation and invited the outdoor industry to contribute to public-private partnerships to help foster a next generation who cares about the outdoors. I'll be pleased when I begin to see more leaders within the fitness industry place the same importance on the outdoors. In the meantime, I believe that each of us can begin to make a difference in the lives of the people within our own circle of influence.

IMPORTANT!

"...the future of our industry AND the future of our nation's public lands depend on reconnecting people—especially our young people—to the outdoors," said Jennifer Mull, Chairman of the Outdoor Industry Association (OIA). [18]

Review

Multiple Choice

Complete the sentence by selecting the correct term or phrase.

1. Which of the following is not a hurdle to wellness?

    a. Digital distraction
    b. Good nutrition
    c. Mental health disorders
    d. Sedentary lifestyle

2. The disorder that refers to a wide array of behavioral problems that stem from not spending enough time outdoors.

    a. Natural distraction disorder
    b. Seasonal affective disorder
    c. Monkey mind
    d. Nature deficit disorder

3. Which of the following is one way to combat things like depression, disengagement from nature, and poor performance in school?

    a. Get children to interact with the outdoors
    b. Encourage children and adults to embrace an outdoor lifestyle
    c. Emphasize free outdoor play
    d. All of the above

4. Nature deficit disorder affects only children, true or false?

    a. True
    b. False

5. Free outdoor play, especially in natural surroundings, has been suggested by some as a way to decrease child obesity, true or false?

a. True

b. False

6. Spending too much time on a digital device can contribute to a sedentary lifestyle and even mental health conditions, true or false?

a. True

b. False

7. According to author Tri Robinson, one of the main drivers of poverty on the planet is childhood obesity, true or false?

a. True

b. False

The Role of Sol Guide Method

Sedentary lifestyle and obesity, mental health disorders, digital distraction, and nature deficit disorders—these are the four challenges that I tailor my outdoor fitness retreats to treat. You may find that you and your clients struggle with additional obstacles to living a vibrant and healthy lifestyle. One thing I'm sure we all share in common is that the demands of modern living can suck the sense of being on an instinctive, wild adventure right out of our every day experience. Leading an outdoor fitness retreat is one way to harness the power of the outdoors and help others live a naturally healthy lifestyle.

According to American Sports Data, Inc. and the International Healthy, Racquet & Sportsclub Association, "between 1990 and 2001, the number of health club members in the U.S. has shot from 20.7 million to 33.8 million, a dramatic 63% increase. Yet their research goes on to further point out that this represents only 13% - 14% of the total U.S. adult population."[19] Fast forward to 2017 and health club and studio membership in the U.S. grew by 33% since 2008—but one in four Americans remained sedentary.[20]

The gym membership data cited above tells us a few things, that 1) population growth is contributing to increases in health club memberships, and 2) the majority of people need more than a gym membership to motivate them to make the time to exercise and stay fit, and 3) one out of every five people in the U.S. are not influenced to join a gym by the prospects of acquiring fewer chronic illnesses and enjoying a longer lifespan.

We want to remain relevant in the effort to make people healthier. To succeed we, as mind/body professionals, must evolve. Continuing to sell one-hour workouts in gyms covered in noisy TV's and electric movement machines may not be the best long-term solution, especially when you consider the four main challenges discussed earlier in this chapter.

How do we help more people connect to their bodies, the planet, and really make a difference in the lives of our communities? As an industry, how do we move the conversation beyond gym and health club membership? How do we expand the scope of our practice when the industry's major certifying bodies restrict our practice to the indoors? The answers to these questions, for me, was found in listening to my clients and responding to their needs. By incorporating my passion for outdoor adventure and my former career experience organizing research expeditions as a wildlife biologist, I was able to craft highly customized and effective outdoor fitness retreats that literally changed my clients lives.

According to the 2018 Physical Activity Council Participation Report, interest in activities has started moving toward outdoor recreation. Their research indicated that the top aspirational activity for all age segments was going outside, and, having a partner to explore outdoors with (or not) played a bigger role in their decision than having the time to do it. [21] I've seen the magic that happens to people in the outdoors as they apply their gym-earned fitness to a real world setting. That magic is the fuel that keeps my fire burning. Once my clients feel the rejuvenation that comes through outdoor adventure, I know they're going to go hiking, stand up paddling, and cycling again without me. And that's fantastic! That's when I know I've done my job. I've gifted someone the joy of movement that led me to this profession in the first place.

Sol Guide Method provides you with the tools to expand your services beyond the gyms and indoor studios and into 'Mother Nature's Gym.' As your programming grows to include outdoor activities, you will effectively increase the overall health and well-being of your clients and your community—and create an additional revenue stream for your practice at the same time.

There are essentially three major components to my Sol Guide Method: body, mind, and nature. I'm sure you've seen some combination of these three terms and concepts before. With this course, I'll explore and share with you how to combine these three elements to create your own outdoor fitness adventure:

- **Body.** Simple strength training, yoga, and mat Pilates sequences that can be performed in any setting, using only 'Mother Nature's Gym.'
- **Mind.** Techniques that train and quiet the mind during an outdoor fitness retreat, including guided visualizations, breathing exercises, and a variety of moving meditations.
- **Nature.** Outdoor recreation activities such as hiking, biking, and stand up paddling that improve overall fitness and provide a fun, safe, and challenging fitness adventure.

We've covered a lot of information. Now take a few minutes to add variety to your study with a few learning activities.

Word Search

Search up, down, forward, backward, and on the diagonal to find and circle the hidden words in the puzzle.

```
M  Q  B  L  S  W  D  A  R  X  H  V  B  Y  S  A  T  T
Z  K  Z  I  Z  S  R  F  U  E  E  B  A  G  T  Q  S  R
C  H  I  F  S  A  F  E  N  F  A  A  L  A  A  D  S  A
F  Y  L  E  G  H  O  V  L  Y  L  I  A  V  N  Z  V  I
J  U  Z  S  K  G  B  X  Q  W  T  M  N  A  D  Z  R  N
E  J  N  T  K  T  U  B  N  I  H  X  C  C  U  X  T  I
X  B  L  Y  P  I  L  A  T  E  S  T  E  X  P  M  T  N
F  F  D  L  M  E  D  I  T  A  T  I  O  N  P  R  Y  G
Q  X  Y  E  H  L  G  D  H  H  O  R  H  O  A  C  K  R
B  R  E  A  T  H  I  N  G  I  U  E  P  E  D  R  X  L
S  T  R  E  N  G  T  H  W  K  T  J  I  N  D  T  V  T
Q  S  T  W  V  R  F  H  E  I  D  U  V  D  L  C  I  X
B  I  T  A  X  U  K  U  L  N  O  V  C  U  E  J  H  S
I  I  G  R  I  B  N  R  L  G  O  E  Y  R  S  A  G  I
Y  A  K  O  E  C  S  L  N  G  R  N  X  A  N  V  M  Q
B  O  M  I  N  S  H  A  E  D  J  A  N  N  J  Y  J  V
L  W  G  B  N  G  S  I  S  L  U  T  L  C  Z  M  U  C
U  E  I  A  Z  G  F  C  S  A  B  E  A  E  V  C  P  U
```

BALANCE	
BIKING	QIGONG
BREATHING	REJUVENATE
ENDURANCE	SAFE
FUN	STANDUPPADDLE
HEALTH	STRENGTH
HIKING	STRESS
LIFESTYLE	TAICHI
MEDITATION	TRAINING
OUTDOOR	WELLNESS
PILATES	YOGA

Multiple Choice

Complete the sentence by selecting the correct term or phrase.
1. Excessive fatness defined as body weight in excess of biological needs.

    a. Diabetes
    b. Obesity
    c. Hypertension
    d. Sedentary lifestyle

2. Normal blood pressure is classified as _____.

    a. Less than 100/100
    b. Less than 120-140/80-90
    c. Less than 160/100
    d. Less than 120/80

3. Which of the following is NOT generally directly linked to obesity.

    a. Stroke
    b. Diabetes
    c. Hyperopia
    d. Hypertension

4. People who are overweight are at increased risk of stroke, which is _____.

    a. A condition characterized by inadequate production of use of insulin
    b. A sudden, focal interruption of cerebral fluid flow that causes a neurologic deficit
    c. Body weight in excess of biological needs
    d. An elevation of blood pressure, especially the diastolic pressure

5. The effects of this type of disorder include a disengagement from nature, attention disorders, depression, and poor performance in school/work.

    a. Nature deficit disorder
    b. Digital distraction
    c. Sedentary lifestyle
    d. Obesity

Matching

Match the list of diagnosable mental health disorders to the appropriate classification.

Diagnosable Mental Health Disorders

_____ post-traumatic stress disorder (PTSD), generalized anxiety, and phobias

_____ antisocial personality disorder, avoidance personality disorder, borderline personality disorder

_____ unipolar depression, bipolar depression

_____ anorexia nervosa, bulimia nervosa, binge eating disorder

Classification

1. Anxiety Disorders
2. Personality Disorders
3. Depression
4. Eating Disorders

Fill in the Blank

Write the word that fits with the sentence in the available spaces below. Not all terms will be used.

_____, or the overuse of electronic media, has been linked to the increase of _____ lifestyles and anxiety disorders. This extensive use of media has been shown to _____ and decrease _____, which leads to reduced levels of _____ One way to combat the ill effects of this phenomenon is to encourage clients to unplug, get outside, and _____.

productivity	digital distraction
increase stress	concentration
exercise	sedentary
seratonin	oxytocin

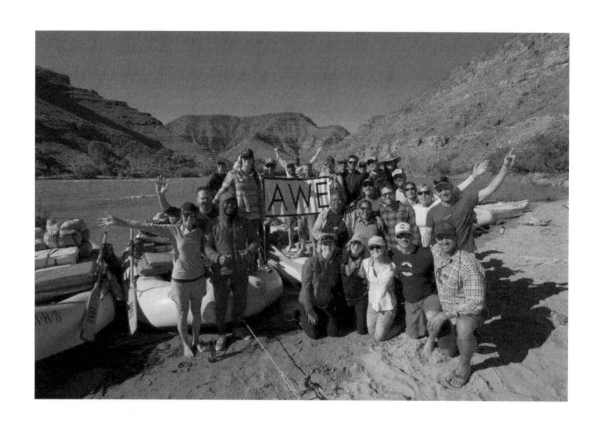

ADVENTURES IN MOTHER NATURE'S GYM

PART TWO
MOTHER NATURE'S GYM

"Man must go back to Nature for information."

– THOMAS PAINE[22]

Nature - The Outdoor Gym

Exercising outdoors plays a crucial role in my personal fitness practice, my lifestyle, and my happiness. It is also foundational to the Sol Guide Method I utilize to create outdoor fitness retreats for my clients, and which I'll share with this course. You'll see that the outdoors appears as a common thread throughout this book.

Whether it was completing my first open water swim while training for a triathlon, skiing down a steep mountainside of deep powdery snow, or stand up paddling in awe of the Pacific Ocean among mating dolphins, life for me has been one amazing outdoor adventure after another.

The ceiling lifted off of my career limitations once my clients started hiring me to train and guide them on their own "bucket list adventures." I extended my gym walls to include 'Mother Nature's Gym' and there was no turning back. Soon I was leading trips to hike the Inca Trail to Machu Picchu, Peru and exploring labyrinthine slot canyons in Southern Utah's National Parks.

I watched as clients applied the strength they had so carefully developed indoors to the unexpected challenges of the outdoors. As they conquered their fears and freed themselves of the shackles of the status quo I began to see nature as the great equalizer and a necessary component of our health and well being as a human family.

In this course you will find a unique learning environment that is effective, efficient, and fun. Once you complete your study and begin leading your own outdoor fitness retreats I hope you'll share this method with other fitness professionals. Together we can make a difference and enhance the world's mind/body/nature connection!

Fitness Settings

I mentioned the fitness gimmicks earlier in the course, and we all know that for a program to have the power to change a person's lifestyle it has to be engaging, fun, and lasting. Gimmicks are none of the above. When I wrote *Adventures in MOTHER NATURE'S GYM*, I knew it had to be engaging, fun, and lasting, but I also knew it had to be grounded in science. While I won't go into detail on the readily available research that explains how physical activity benefits physical and mental health, I do want to look at the specific science behind what makes an outdoor fitness retreat different from the typical fitness session.

Think about a time when you were outside and everything—the scenery, the air, and your body—seemed perfect. There really is something about being out in nature that just *feels* good.

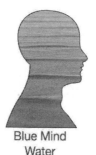
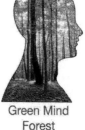
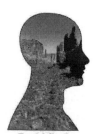

Blue Mind
Water | Green Mind
Forest | Red Mind
Desert

While feeling good is reason enough for extending fitness programming into the outdoor arena, there is a growing body of scientific evidence that explains why being outdoors is so good for us. This new field of study is collectively called neuroconservation and includes research that focuses on why being near water, the forest, or the desert can make our minds and bodies happy. The ultimate objective of neuroconservation is that if we can understand what happens when our brain meets the outdoors we just may be able to use that information to help drive public policy and influence public health for the better.[23]

In this section of the course I'll explore a few of the different mindsets that have been coined from the study of what happens to the mind and body while engaged in nature. In addition I'll share some of the learning activities and meditations that I use during my own outdoor fitness retreats. The three mindsets are Blue Mind, Green Mind, and Red, or Desert Mind.

Blue Mind

What is it about water that makes it so critical to human existence? The comprised of about 80% water. Each water molecule in your body has oceanic realm in the past. Water in our bodies may have once flowed in as vapor suspended in clouds, or been locked in glacial ice. All life depe in some way.

One of the scientists leading the conversation about humans and water is scientist Wallace J. Nichols, research associate at the California Academy of Sciences. In his book Blue Mind, he presents the surprising science that shows how being near, in, on, or under water can "Make you happier, healthier, more connected, and better at what you do." How does all of this "feeling good" happen? Good question!

When you're close to water, your brain releases cascades of the feel-good chemicals dopamine, serotonin, and oxytocin. Once you step into the water, the pressure of the water against your body balances the stress hormone catecholamine, which regulates function of the arteries. During immersion, the body sends a signal to balance catecholamine levels, which produces a relaxation effect similar to that achieved during meditation. In other words, just being in the water can cause a feeling of relaxation.[24]

Regular exercise is associated with the number of new neurons in the hippocampus area of the brain (the area associated with memory and learning). More neurons mean greater cognitive function.

Here comes the cool part: the way you move your body in the water during swimming—timing the breath, moving the legs at one rhythm and the arms at another—is completely different than the way you move on land. The complex coordination of the swim stroke requires you to use your mind's cognitive functioning to swim. Now science has proven that the combination of cognitive functioning and aerobic exercise creates the greatest amount of cognitive reserve - literally the mind's resilience to damage of the brain.[25]

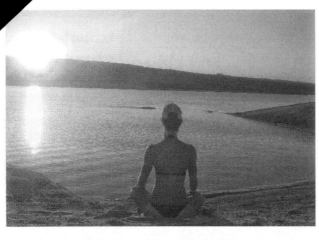

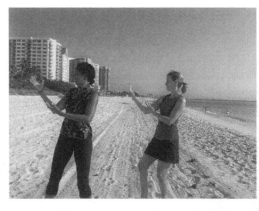

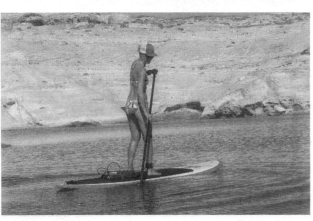

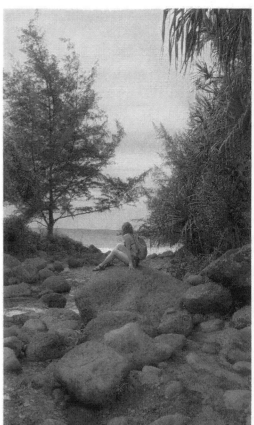

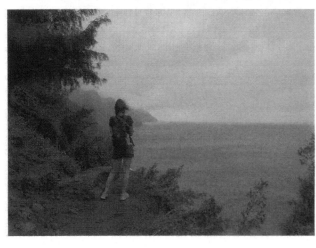

Word Search

Search up, down, forward, backward, and on the diagonal to find and circle the hidden words in the puzzle.

```
R  E  L  A  X  A  T  I  O  N  C  L  T  U
Q  N  V  D  W  F  B  R  A  I  N  X  A  C
H  I  P  P  O  C  A  M  P  U  S  O  A  D
A  W  Y  K  G  G  B  O  Y  R  S  T  M  O
I  A  C  N  P  K  X  N  E  Q  E  R  M  P
A  T  C  M  Y  Y  O  S  T  C  N  E  I  A
Q  E  I  F  T  J  I  N  H  I  D  M  V  M
H  R  Z  O  W  L  W  O  J  I  M  X  Y  I
A  A  C  V  I  H  L  R  T  E  X  M  N  N
N  I  P  E  E  A  B  A  R  F  H  C  K  E
N  P  N  P  M  T  T  S  M  E  M  O  R  Y
H  C  E  I  Y  I  I  I  L  Q  U  T  J  C
E  J  N  E  O  O  R  H  Y  T  H  M  I  C
I  E  Q  N  N  S  E  R  O  T  O  N  I  N
```

BRAIN
CATECHOLAMINE
DOPAMINE
HAPPY
HIPPOCAMPUS
IMMERSION
MEDITATION

MEMORY
OXYTOCIN
RELAXATION
RESILIENCE
RHYTHMIC
SEROTONIN
WATER

Blue Mind in Action

You may want to incorporate activities designed to help your clients access their Blue Mind state and notice the feelings of tranquility that come with water activities.

Here are a couple of activities you can use any time you are incorporating water into your outdoor adventure.

Blue Marble Game

One of my favorite things to do on stand up paddle retreats or hikes through rivers is play the Blue Marble Game, created by marine biologist and economist Wallace J. Nichols. I love the game in its simplicity, in its ability to remind us that this blue planet we call home is distinguished from all others because of our water. It's fun to send my clients—especially the kids—home with a little token from our day spent adventuring together. I've had guests—and even other guides—tell me they still have their blue marble several years after I've gifted one to them.

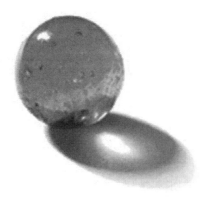

The real beauty of the Blue Marble Game is in its intention of spreading an attitude of gratitude around the globe. I still remember the first time I received my own Blue Marble from 'J,' during a keynote he gave in Veracruz, Mexico for an event with the

Adventure Travel Trade Association in 2011. He brought the room to tears with this one simple gesture and I've seen it do the same with my own clients ever since. There are only five rules to playing the game:

1. The marble must be blue (order a set with your own branded pass-along cards at www.bluemarbles.org).
2. When you receive a blue marble, give it away to someone as a token of gratitude.
3. Ask the person to hold the marble to the sky as they look into it. Explain that this is what the Earth looks like from 1,000,000 miles away.
4. Invite the person to hold the marble to their heart as they think of a person who actively cares for the planet.
5. Share your story with the world (however you like – in an Instagram or Tweet, for example).

MEL SAYS

Families are a joy to guide on fitness retreats. On one Southern Utah hiking adventure I guided a family of three generations: a grandma and grandpa from Washington, D.C. with their daughter, her husband, and two little boys from San Francisco, California. We went to Zion National Park in Utah and hiked part of the Zion Narrows, formed entirely by the erosion forces of the Virgin River, and talked about the importance of the river to the Native American people and early Mormon Pioneer settlers. Standing on the banks of the river, we played the Blue Marble Game. The three-year-old prized his blue marble. He clutched it tightly in his little hand and fell asleep with it on our drive back to the hotel. His mother thanked me and told me she knew it would live in his box of treasures at home.

ACTIVITY

Guided Imagery

This type of meditation is called guided imagery and is a great tool to use with clients with a high stress level or who simply want to relax and enjoy their water surroundings on a deeper level. When leading guided imagery, use words to create and hold a picture and sensory association in the mind.

I once used this meditation with four busy adventure travel journalists while stand up paddling at Lake Powell on a magical fall day. They described the result as having "all types of Zen restored."

Start by inviting clients to find a relaxing position, either lying down on paddleboards, on the ground, or sitting comfortably. Instruct them close their eyes, clear their minds and begin to focus their attention on their breathing. Their breathing should be slow and gentle as they imagine the touch, sight, smell, and sound of the words you say. Say each word out loud and leave enough time to experience the sensory stimulation that can accompany each word.

Say aloud:

Flow	Lake
Soft	Pond
Wet	Drink
Hot	Cool
Shallow	Brackish
Cold	Turbulent
Current	Smooth
Ripple	Murky
Pool	Clear
Ocean	Deep

ACTIVITY

Connecting With Water

To do this activity you'll need a body of water, preferably from a natural source, but a nice water feature will do too.

- Turn off your cell phone
- Set a timer for 10 minutes
- Sit down or lie next to, on, or in the water
- Close your eyes and focus on your breathing
- Allow yourself to just be quiet and attentive to the sound, smell, touch, and sight of the water and your own body
- After 10 minutes, take a moment to write down all of the ways you experienced water using your five senses

You likely have some personal connections to water. Use your experiences and connections to create your own Blue Mind activities.

Blue Mind - Try it Now

There are so many ways one can connect and help others connect with water. Take some time now to brainstorm ways you can connect with water. Think also about a game you can play with your clients to help them make a connection with their own blue minds.

What is one way you can connect with your 'Blue Mind?'

Think of a game or meditation exercise you could play with clients to help them connect with water. Make sure to include as many tactile, sensory details as possible – write down what it smells, tastes, looks and feels like to experience this game and tap into that Blue Mind state.

Green Mind

The Slow Movement hit mainstream media in November 2012 when journalist Florence Williams wrote "The Nature Cure," published in *Outside Magazine*.[26] Williams traveled to Japan to investigate why the government invested millions of dollars into developing walking paths in cities and forests and actively promotes the health benefits of walking outside.

Williams found her answer. Research had indicated that walking in a green forest decreases physiological measures like heart rate and blood pressure. She joined University of Chiba scientist Yoshifumi Miyazaki for a clinical comparison of the brain activity and vital signs of 12 male college students during a walk in a forest versus a walk in an urban setting.

REMEMBER!

The sympathetic nervous system controls the physiological reactions to threats (fight or flight response). Quieting the sympathetic nervous system and making the shift to the parasympathetic nervous system allows the body to relax.

Williams was not an official participant in the study, but she did have her vital signs measured. She learned that when she was walking calmly in the forest, oxyhemoglobin concentrations in the prefrontal cortex of her brain declined, showing that her sympathetic nervous system had gotten a restorative break. Her systolic blood pressure had dropped six points by the end of the forest walk, whereas it rose six points during the city walk.[27]

Fill in the Blank

Fill in the blanks in the paragraph below using the list of words provided. Not all words will be used.

The country of _____ has invested millions of dollars developing _____ paths in cities and forests. The benefits of walking outside in a forest include _____ systolic blood pressure. Walking in a _____ setting stimulates the _____ nervous system to _____.

South Korea
increased
parasympathetic
relax
lower
walking
calm
Germany

stimulating
blue
prancercising
heighten
decreased
running
sympathetic
Japan

Green Mind in Action

I've found that using terms like 'mindfulness' or 'meditation' can scare some people off. If you're not sure that your clients are open to a meditation session, you can still help them get their daily dose of 'nature cure' by guiding them through some very simple observation exercises. These exercises can help even the most uptight urban dwellers access the much needed relaxation benefits of spending time outdoors.

In this section I've shared two of the relaxation and mindfulness activities I've seen work well with my clients on outdoor fitness retreats: Meet the Five Senses and Guided Visualization.

ACTIVITY

Meet the Five Senses

One of the most inspiring principles I've learned from my Navajo friends is that nature actually has something to tell us too—it's not meant to be just a one-sided conversation. Navajo children learn from a very young age to take cues from nature. I suppose this is something all of our primal ancestors knew how to do instinctively. When I spend several days camping in the wilderness or unplugging on an outdoor vacation, I can feel myself get into that space. It's so…. natural and instinctive, really! When I'm living every day life in the city, I have to work a little harder to get to a park or grove of trees, to turn off my mobile device and sit still long enough to access that space of being in tune with my surroundings.

The real beauty of Meet the Five Senses rests in its simplicity. There are four simple guidelines to playing this game:

1. Hike, bike, or stand up paddle your way to a beautiful outdoor setting
2. Instruct the group to use the five senses to observe their surroundings
3. Invite everyone to find his or her own sweet spot to sit and notice nature
4. Call the group together after 5-10 minutes to share their findings

ACTIVITY

Guided Visualization

The next progression from guided imagery is visualization. During this exercise you guide others through an experience with their senses through the use of phrases that stimulate memory and associated responses.

Follow these steps to guide your clients through a visualization exercise:

1. Choose your favorite outdoor activity to access a beautiful outdoor setting – kayaking, biking, spelunking, whatever it is you've centered your retreat around.
2. Keeping the group together, instruct them to sit or lie still with their eyes closed.
3. Begin with 5-10 cycles of deep relaxing breaths, melting into the floor or the ground with each breath.
4. Invite the group to imagine the sight, touch, taste, smell, and sound of each phrase as you read it out loud. Be sure to speak slowly, allowing a few seconds between phrases to give everyone ample time to access the memory. I've shared a few of my favorites here, but feel free to create your own list of relaxation phrases.

The feel of wet grass under your feet in the early morning
The smell of a pine forest
The sight of an open mountain meadow
The sounds of jungle animals
The taste of a fresh picked apple
The touch of your favorite plant
The color of your favorite flower
The smell of smoke on the breeze
The sound of night falling on a summer evening

The Power of Wilderness

One of my favorite authors is the late Edward Abbey, who wrote about my homeland in the desert southwest. The excerpt below is from his book *The Journey Home* and influenced my thinking as I was formulating my business Sol Fitness Adventures back in 2004.

"The wildest animal I know is you, gentle reader, with this helpless book clutched in your claws…we need wilderness because we are wild animals. Every man needs a place where he can go to go crazy in peace. Every Boy Scout troop needs a forest to get lost, miserable, and starving in. Even the maddest murderer of the sweetest wife should get a chance to run for the hills. If only for the sport of it. For the terror, the delirium…Because we need brutality and raw adveture. What makes life in our cities at once still tolerable, exciting, and stimulating is the existence of an alternative option, whether exercised or not, whether even appreciated or not, of a radically different mode of being out there in the forests, on the lakes and rivers, up in the mountains… To be alive is to take risks; to be always safe and secure is death."[28]

Green Mind - Try it Now

Making a connection with green spaces helps quiet the mind and relax the body. Take some time to think about how you can connect with your 'green mind' more often, and how you can help others connect with the green spaces on your retreat or in their own community to improve their health and well-being.

JOURNAL ENTRY - GREEN MIND

What is one way you can connect with your green mind?

Think of a game you can play with clients to help them connect with green spaces. Specifically, what elements of a forest, mountain, jungle, or meadow can you use to help your client focus their attention and be present?

Desert Mind

Confession time. Red, or Desert Mind, is the body-mind according to . . . me, the Sol Fitness Adventures outdoor fitness guide. I lead the majority of my outdoor fitness retreats in the arid, vast desert landscapes of the Mojave Desert, Great Basin, and Colorado Plateau. Aside from several of my favorite non-fiction books written by well-respected desert-dwellers, I have not found much scientific research that details what's going on physiologically in these desert environments. I suppose the neuroscientists just haven't made it to my neck of the woods in the Southwest yet. If you meet one who's interested, send them my way!

I tend to gravitate to the desert more than any other landscape, perhaps because I was born in Utah and my great, great grandparents settled the extreme southwest corner of the state, which happens to be in the Mojave Desert. Before my grandfather, a retired dairy farmer and horseman, died at the age of 92 he put his hands on my head and reminded me that I have the red sands of St. George coursing through my veins and DNA. I was living in Washington, D.C. at the time, something he couldn't understand given my love of my desert homeland. Like my grandfather, I had come to understand, even find solace in, the solitude found in the desert. The late Minister William Edelin, based in the Coachella Valley in California, wrote this of the desert:

"The desert reduces everything to essentials, to the basics of whitened

bone. The desert, perhaps more than any other place on earth,

speaks of silence, simplicity and solitude. The desert calls to men

and women who being wasted away by the stress, confusion and

anxieties of city life, yearn for a spiritual retreat, an escape from

the demon time, the clock and the calendar that so enslave us."[29]

More than any other location, it is the desert landscapes of the Four Corners Region that my own clients have requested I take them on their customized outdoor fitness retreats. While part of that is certainly because it's the place I call home and that I know the best; the other part, the one that is often more difficult for them to articulate, is that they feel drawn to the desert out of their deep inner desire to find a place of peace and solitude. It's as if the simplicity of the desert, described by Mr. Edelin, beckons to them when they are finally ready to escape the noise.

Without the breadth of scientific facts to share, like those found in the Blue Mind and Green Mind sections, I've chosen to take a deep dive into the more esoteric realm with Desert Mind. Here I share what I've learned from the healers I've met through my own adventures around the world. You'll find definitions and references to the concepts introduced here in the 'key terms' section on the next few pages.

Astrophysics – The search to understand the universe and our place in it. Key questions asked include: 1) How does the universe work, 2) How did we get here, and 3) Are we alone?

Alpha brain wave – Alpha waves occur at a frequency of 8 to 12 cycles per second in a regular rhythm. They are present only when you are awake but have your eyes closed. Usually they disappear when you open your eyes.[30]

Chakra – "Padmas" in Sanskrit. Cerebrospinal centers composed of prana (life force). Awakening the spirituality of the cerebrospinal centers is the sacred goal of the yogi. There are six spinal centers (medullary, cervical, dorsal, lumbar, sacral, and coccygeal plexuses).[31]

Electroencephalogram (EEG) – Measures abnormalities in brain waves and brain electrical activity. Performed in a laboratory using two electrodes with small metal discs attached to the skull. The electrodes measure the electrical changes that take place in brain cells.

OM – "Aum" in Sanskrit, the ancient language of India. The cosmic vibratory power behind all atomic energies. The Creative Word and witness of Divine Presence. The sound heard in meditation during Kriya Yoga.[32]

Indian Rishis – Refers to the wise 'sages' of India. The Gods revealed the Vedas (truths of the eternal creator and creation) to the rishi, which became the foundation of Indian civilization. The rishis practiced Vedic Yoga, the oldest of yoga practices.[33]

Pachamama – In Incan (Peruvian natives) culture, means earth goddess, earth mother, Mother Earth.[34]

Schumann Resonance – Electromagnetic waves that exist in the cavity between the earth's crust and the inner edge of the ionosphere at 55 km up. Seemingly related to electrical activity in the atmosphere, particularly during a lightning storm. Occur at several frequencies. Detected by physicists Schumann and Konig in 1954.[35]

While there may not be a depth of scientific research specific to our physiologic response to the desert, some science *does* exist concerning a measurable frequency of the earth's vibrations. The magnetic field of the Earth has a frequency of 7.83 Hz called the Schumann Resonance. This is the same frequency that the Indian Rishis called "OM." This frequency has been associated with high levels of hypnotizability, meditation, increased human growth hormone (HGH) levels, and increased cerebral blood flows.

The human body is a conglomerate of frequencies. Alpha brain waves—those associated with relaxed and effortless wakefulness—were originally set at a frequency of 7.5 – 12.5 Hz, [36] though research data varies, citing frequencies between 8 – 13 Hz[37] and even 9 – 14 Hz. Interestingly, theta brainwaves are measured at a frequency between 5 and 8 Hz and are associated with the free flow of creative ideas that occur during automatic, repetitive tasks, such as showering or driving on the freeway.[38]

Are you still with me? What I'm getting at is that the frequency of the earth and that of the two most relaxed and creative – yet awake – states of the human mind occur within the same range of frequencies. What do these numbers and frequencies mean? Is there a correlation between our blue planet's magnetic resonance and the human alpha and theta brain waves? Does the human body/mind need the earth to be healthy, or are the similar frequencies of the earth and the brain mere coincidence? To ask the question another way, are the increasing rates of occurrence of mental illness related to extreme cases of nature deprivation?

I don't think it is a stretch to realize intuitively that we need nature to be healthy!

It's interesting that the root chakra, the 1st chakra that grounds us, is closest to the ground. The color assigned to the root chakra is the color red - red like the Navajo sandstone layer of the Mojave Desert in my beloved Zion National Park. I see the grounding effects that nature has on my clients. Many of them come on a personal journey of healing, discovery, and rejuvenation and go home looking 10 years younger. While I like to think that my techniques help guide them in their journey, I know there's a magic happening from being 'on the land,' as American Indians call it, that I am only a witness to.

Rachel Carson was a marine biologist and author who is credited for bringing environmental concerns to the forefront of the American consciousness. The following is an excerpt from her book *The Sense of Wonder*:

"Those who dwell...among the beauties and mysteries of the

earth are never alone or weary of life. Whatever the vexations or

concerns of their personal lives, their thoughts can find paths that

lead to inner contentment and to renewed excitement in living.

Those who contemplate the beauty of the earth find reserves of

strength that will endure as long as life lasts...there is something

infinitely healing in the repeated refrains of nature – the assurance

that dawn comes after night, and spring after the winter."[39]

Desert Mind in Action

I find it easiest to tap into my alpha and beta mind frequencies when I exercise, and if I couple that with being outdoors, especially in the desert, those mind states are magnified. My alone-ness is no longer loneliness, but becomes a comfortable, even welcome solitude. When I guide clients on an outdoor fitness retreat I find that there are a few emotions that often accompany that experience – feelings of solitude, love, and support.

ACTIVITY

Solitude

Between work, social, family or community responsibilities and the constant need to be 'plugged in,' I have to work hard now to get meaningful solitude. I love to be quiet and read a book just as much as I enjoy being with people, but nothing compares to the feeling of being in the outdoors, alone.

JOURNAL ENTRY - SOLITUDE ACTIVITY

How often are you alone, unplugged, and still enough to really hear your own thoughts and intuition?

ACTIVITY

Supported

There have been many times when I'm guiding that I actually feel the power of Mother Nature supporting me in my work. Whether I'm caught in an unexpected thunderstorm in a slot canyon or helping a client overcome a physical challenge or paralyzing fear, I have literally felt 'Pachamama' energize and sustain me in what I need to do. This may sound kind of 'woo-woo' or mystical to the uninitiated, but I suspect that some of you have experienced the same thing. If you haven't, I suspect that someday you will!

JOURNAL ENTRY - SUPPORTED ACTIVITY

What makes you feel supported?

ACTIVITY

Loved

If love is an emotion that heals, calms, attracts, and brings us back to ourselves, then love is certainly an emotion I have felt in the outdoors. I believe that if what we seek is a greater ability to love others, to feel the love of the Universe, God, or the Creator - whatever that means to you – and to connect with our essential life force, then nurturing a connection to the outdoors is a critical ingredient.

Facing fears in the outdoors can be a metaphor for facing our fears in love. When things appear too daunting we may choose to avoid the situation, turn away from it, and close ourselves off to the experience. But to overcome the fear or rise to the challenge we have to face it and remain open to the possibility that we just might succeed. Being with Mother Nature can teach powerful lessons in vulnerability, a necessary ingredient for creating intimacy in our relationships.

JOURNAL ENTRY - LOVED ACTIVITY

What makes you feel loved? Is there a specific outdoor setting where you've been able to experience your essential life force?

The Power of Awe

An entire branch of neuroscientists actively study what happens in the human brain when we experience something that creates in us a sense of awe, a feeling of reverential respect mixed with fear or wonder. Stimuli may include the sound of a beautiful melody, the sight of a spectacular landscape, even an act of athletic prowess. "Awe happens when people encounter a vast and unexpected stimulus, something that makes them feel small…awe prompts people to redirect concern away from the self and toward everything else. And three-quarters of the time, it's elicited by nature."[40]

A client in Santa Barbara gifted me one of my favorite writings on awe in the form of a newspaper clipping. In the article, the late Minister William Edelen captured the essence of the emotion awe when he said, "Our sense of the sacred is awakened when we use the mountain as the focus of our meditations…we respond with awe and wonder and a sound of joy pours forth from our throat that we cannot hold back. 'Ah,' we say, and it is in that 'Ah' that the depth of our spirit comes forth and we are awake as we sanctify the moment and the place where we are."[41]

It was actually the concept of awe—and my own timely encounter with the emotion—that compelled me to make the edits required to re-publish this course. In case it's been a while since you've had an awe moment I'll share mine, and hope that it inspires you to pick up something that you've been wanting to accomplish.

In 2016 and 2017 I worked as editor and project manager on *The Outsider* by KUHL, an ambitious storytelling project by a leading outdoor and lifestyle clothing company. Through my work I crossed paths with other groups and individuals working to improve health using the outdoors. One of these people was Stacy Bare. A veteran who worked for Sierra Club at the time and an athlete for The North Face, Stacy leads veterans on skiing and climbing adventures back to the countries where they once fought wars as a way to help heal old wounds and gain closure.

Stacy, it turned out, was scheming a river trip with Candra Canning of Live Bright Now and Steve Markle, the V.P. of Marketing of O.A.R.S. rafting. I'd met Steve and his wife in 2010 while hiking a glacier in Switzerland during the annual Adventure Travel Trade Association Summit, a global gathering of professionals who serve adventurous travelers, like I do with Sol Fitness Adventures.

Stacy and Steve invited me to attend their 2017 Expedition Colloquium, a four-day river trip through one of the most remote areas in the lower 48 – Desolation Canyon on the Green River, Utah. The trip had three objectives: 1) to brainstorm ways to create public policy to support veterans with government-funded outdoor-based programs, 2) to give all of us the chance to unplug from our digital devices for four days so that we could have an experience of awe for ourselves, and 3) to create a short documentary film about the healing that one veteran river guide in particular, Garret Eaton, has found being on the river.[42]

For four spectacularly unplugged days our floating think tank of 20 engaged in in-depth conversation about our work in the world and how each of us harnesses the power of nature and adventure to transform the various populations we serve. "Finally!" I thought. There were professionals from non-profits, State and Federal Government, and private sector. Even Silicon Valley was represented, as the founders of the biggest technology companies of our time grapple with the responsibility of creating a digitally dependent society that is addicted to smart phones. We immersed ourselves in the wild, settling into deeply personal conversations of our encounters with Mother Nature, our own healing journeys, and what makes a person resilient. Gathered around the fire each night we acted out skits and presented our ideas of how to make spending time in the outdoors a more conscious and deliberate aspect of American life.

The river supplied awe in ample measure, and the trip was the spark I needed to pick up my writing and republish *Adventures in MOTHER NATURE'S GYM*. Finally the tide of awareness has turned. If nature has the power to heal those stricken with the battle scars of war, abuse, and addiction, imagine what it can do for the general population as a preventative approach to health and wellness. While I have a great deal of respect for the outdoor and adventure travel guides (I am one, after all), I can't think of any group of people better positioned to lead this effort than my own peers in the fitness and mind-body industries.

Desert Mind - Try it Now

Here I invite you to think about how you can connect more deeply with your desert mind. It's alright if you've never been to the desert – how can you apply these thought questions to your own special outdoor places?

JOURNAL ENTRY - DESERT MIND

Think about ways you can connect with your desert mind.

What emotions and insights do you experience when you tap into your alpha and beta mind frequencies?

What type of things can you do to help your clients connect with their 'desert minds?'

Maintaining a Connection to Nature

I learned the hard way what happens when I don't maintain a connection to nature. Can you relate to my experience below?

MEL SAYS

In 2008 I lived and worked in Washington, D.C. For a six-month period I made a mistake common to many young and energetic personal trainers and mind/body professionals – I worked six days a week training an average of 8–10 clients a day in the gym. Not only did I burn out mentally; physically I was run down, depleted, and literally sick. All I wanted to do was to drive to the towering red rock canyon walls of my former home near Zion National Park. If only I could just go sit in the sun—I would feel so much better!

The next day as I lay sick in bed I meditated on Zion. I imagined the warmth of sun on my skin, the sound of quiet, the smell of dry earth, sagebrush, and creosote. I saw the deep red hues of land punctuated by the muddy flash flood waters of the Virgin River. I thought of the countless days walking the river's banks during my three years as a wildlife biologist. Memories of special moments with clients and friends in the canyon swelled my heart and brought tears to my eyes. How I longed to be there in that moment!

I felt better soon enough. But my Zion meditation was the first step in closing the chapter on my seven-year stay in D.C. It was time to go home, time to go to work creating something that others could turn to and simply feel better.

Review

Matching

Match the correct term or phrase to the appropriate space. Not all terms will be used.

awe
neuro-conservation
angst
Blue Mind
spinal cord
dopamine, serotonin, oxytocin
sympathetic nervous system
white mind
caffeine, alcohol, tobacco
catecholamine

1. Research that focuses on why being near water, the forest, or
 the desert can make our minds and bodies happy.

2. This science shows that being near, in, or under water can
make you happier, healthier, and better at what you do.

3. A stress hormone.

4. Feel-good chemicals.

5. Controls your reactions to threats (fight or flight response).

6. A feeling of reverential respect mixed with fear or wonder.

Multiple Choice

Complete each sentence by selecting the correct term or phrase.

1. The objective of the neuro-conservation movement is to _____.

    a. Increase the sales of outdoor adventure equipment
    b. Urge athletes to workout in the outdoors instead of in gyms
    c. Help drive public policy and influence public health for the better
    d. Reduce power consumption

2. In her book The Nature Cure, Florence Williams found scientific support for the idea that walking in _____ decreases physiological measures such as _____.

    a. An urban setting, hear rate, and blood pressure
    b. A green forest, brain function, and metabolism
    c. An urban setting, brain function, and metabolism
    d. A green forest, heart rate, and blood pressure

3. The root chakra is the 1st chakra and keeps us grounded. The color associated with the root chakra is _____.

    a. Red
    b. White
    c. Blue
    d. Green

4. A person who is at great peace when in a forest may connect easily with this category of mindset.

    a. Blue mind
    b. Green mind
    c. Desert mind
    d. None of the above

5. Someone who feels especially connected when on the water has tapped into this category of mind set.

    a. Blue mind
    b. Green mind
    c. Desert mind
    d. None of the above

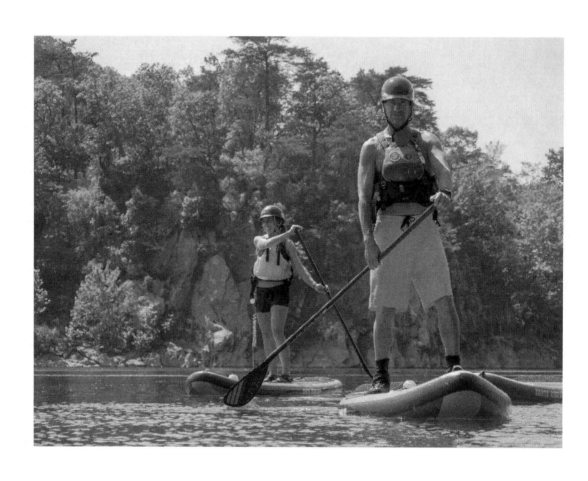

PART THREE
SOL GUIDE METHOD

"We do not run risks acting on our beliefs, but occupy hours each day watching actors who pretend to have adventures, engaged in mock-meaningful action."

– MIHALY CSIKSZENTMIHALYI

Imagine you are at work one day, doing what you do, making things happen...when a stranger approaches you. The stranger says, "Teach me how to do your job in two minutes." First of all, you would probably be irritated that someone interrupted you to make such a ridiculous request. You also might wonder why he wanted to know how to do *your* job. If you truly considered his question, could you really tell the person how to do your job in two minutes? You have dedicated your career to learning how to do things right, how to be efficient, and how to anticipate problems. There is a whole body of knowledge and experience you have that can't be easily translated into words.

Like your work, Sol Guide Method is not a simple prescribed regimen or one-size-fits-all sequence to follow—it is the culmination of a lifetime of personal and professional encounters with fitness and the outdoors. Like old traditions and stories that get passed down, Sol Guide Method is a thought process—a personalized, detail-oriented service that fosters a connection to the body.

You are a dedicated fitness professional with a wealth of knowledge that your clients can benefit from. Once you learn to trust yourself in a variety of settings and be in tune with what you see and feel happening in your client's body and emotions, you can tap into an intuitive flow of exercises that becomes more than just a workout, it becomes a healing experience.

Challenge, Lift, Engage

As you use Sol Guide Method to enhance your practice, keep in mind that the ultimate goal is to challenge the body, lift the spirit, and engage the senses in nature. You can use the thought processes presented in this section as frameworks to guide you as you select from the thousands of exercises you already know and insert that one exercise into the workout that would simply *feel good next*. As you settle into a rhythm of exercise sequencing, assist your client in making the natural transition to being present. Being open to the healing relaxation that movement provides can usher your clients into that hard to reach "flow" state.

What is a "flow" state, you ask? Good question. We'll move on and find out, after some words on healing and a quick review.

IMPORTANT!

A Note on Healing

This book is not intended to make you a "healer." I've sought many a healer in my travels and encountered only a few. I don't claim to be a guru, or that the Sol Guide Method of leading outdoor fitness retreats will heal people. I think we can all agree that the work we do as mind/body professionals—that of helping clients and communities live healthier, happier lives—is restorative; a type of healing if you will. Among us there are healers. We're a group of caring, nurturing people with a genuine desire to serve others. Our intention, combined with a personalized, detail-oriented service, the inherent nurturing power of Mother Nature, and a client who is ready to receive what each retreat and destination has to offer them, can create healing experiences that yield long term benefits.

Fill in the Blank

Enter the appropriate term into the spaces provided. Not all terms will be used.

1. "_____ is more than a generic _____ workout. It is a way of _____."

life   nature   gym   fitness

2. It is important to tap into an intuitive _____ of_____ that becomes _____.

flow   healing   exercise   spirit

3. Our _____ combined with a personalized _____ service, the inherent _____ of _____, and a client who is ready to _____ can be a healing experience.

healing powers   receive   give   Mother Nature   detail-oriented   intention

Flow State

Ask any serious athlete what it feels like to be in "the zone" and they'll describe being fully focused on their activity, with every movement feeling effortless. It is almost an out-of-body experience. It's an incredible feeling. I used to spend hours a day in this state of mind when I was a competitive volleyball and softball player in high school, and later a runner. Now it is a state that I long for and miss feeling on a regular basis. For distance runners, this same state of mind is often called "runner's high."

The "zone" state of mind isn't limited to competitive athletes. Creative people spend time in that state, too. You may have noticed this sensation at work even – when you've been so engaged that the time seemed to just 'fly.' Artists, craftsmen, and writers - they all experience being in the zone...only they don't call it the "zone."

Psychologist Mihaly Csikszentmihaly discovered that when both skill and challenge are high a person can enter a flow channel. Flow is achieved when you're doing something you like to do and you feel two important things simultaneously, 1) arousal – the activity is intriguing and engaging and you are fully immersed mentally, and 2) control – you are in command of your skills and the subject matter.

EXAMPLE

If you consider the Blue Mind, Green Mind, and Desert Mind concepts introduced in Part Three of this course and apply the idea of flow, you can begin to imagine fitness activities in the outdoors where your clients can experience flow in settings that put their minds and bodies at ease:

- Stand up paddle in crystalline water, observing the dolphins swim next to you.
- Hike to the top of a steep cliff, watching the golden eagles riding the wind.
- Strike a yoga pose in the ancient desert where dinosaurs once roamed.

Are you beginning to catch the vision of the kind of variety and outdoor fitness retreats you can create for your clients?

Csikszentmihalyi explains that you can't get into a flow state when you are not completely engaged in something - while sitting on the toilet or watching TV, for example. Doing those mindless activities you may feel like you are "zoning out," but flow state is more like zoning in. You only achieve flow when you're comfortable but not excited, learning while being pushed.[43]

Psychologist, meditation teacher, and author George Mumford helps describe flow by explaining its opposite in his book *The Mindful Athlete: Secrets to Top Performance*. Mumford says, "no matter how strong or skillful you might be, your mind can also impede that talent from being expressed, and it often does so in insidious ways if you don't take care of it... the mind is a muscle. You need to take care of it through daily practice. It's that simple and that profound."[44]

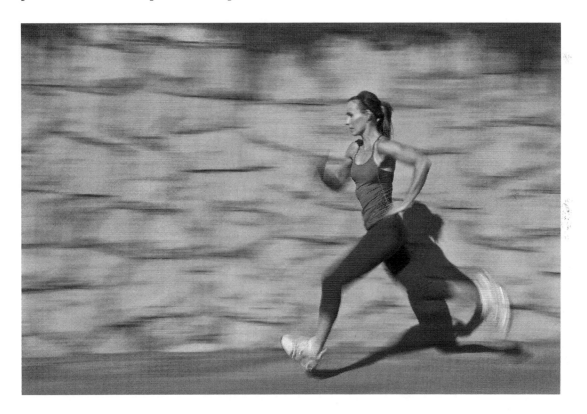

What does flow have to do with creating fitness retreats? Flow is important because the outdoor activities your clients engage in should create feelings of arousal and control. They should be challenging yet enjoyable. If you have guided them to the right activities and they are in the right state of mind, they can tap into that flow channel. You may even witness them experience flow for the first time, which is a thrill as a guide and coach!

Lead your clients on an experiential fitness adventure, one that perfectly highlights their abilities and captures their full attention. Then watch them fall in love with that feeling. It's that feeling that will keep them going back again and again, living an active lifestyle that keeps them healthy and happy.

JOURNAL ENTRY – FLOW

Reflection is an important tool to understand the concepts and ideas presented in this course. Read the following phrases and ponder on what the phrase means to you. This is strictly for you! Think of these journal entries as a place where you can collect your thoughts and the ideas that resonate with you.

Challenge the body
Lift the spirits
Engage the senses in nature
Transition to being present
Be open to healing
Reach the flow state

Sol Guide Method - Body, Mind, and Nature

By now you have probably figured out that Sol Guide Method revolves around three important systems:

- Body
- Mind
- Nature

When combined into an outdoor fitness retreat, body, mind, and nature can create a harmonious, life-changing experience that indoor training programs simply cannot duplicate. In this chapter, I'll explore each of these elements in depth and share how to apply them to building your own retreats.

One of my favorite career highlights was being a Sponsored Athlete for ATHLETA, a Gap Brand, in 2012. That was before Instagram was big and there was no such thing as a paid social media 'influencer.' While I didn't have a large social media following what I did have was credibility and real, on the ground interaction with a lot of influential people. I wrote about one of my favorite fitness adventures in the ATHLETA chi blog. Allow me to share a little walk down that memory lane with an excerpt from The Magic of Bali:

One of my favorite trips was a hiking/stand up paddling adventure

to Bali, Indonesia. I took a yoga session that overlooked the sea

and learned a refreshing way to connect and be present.

I'd heard much about the famed yoga retreats of Bali, and, not a regular

practitioner, welcomed the chance to attend classes with a local teacher,

Ketut Bandiastra Cahya. Ketut never uttered a single 'asana.' His cues were simple, his postures flowed, his message was pure: "Check in with the body. Check in with the emotions. Smile. The purpose of yoga is happiness." The ocean air and jungle melody provided the ideal setting, and I slept easily during the rest phase at each session. I turned myself over to the peace and harmony with welcome surrender...

Years ago I practiced yoga with a shaman in Cusco, Peru, prior to a multi-day Inca Trail trek with several clients. The shaman instructed me to be open to what the Inca Trail had to offer me. I didn't know at the time what he meant, so I approached the challenge with an open mind, and it was there that I learned to 'connect with my adventure...'

The invitation of any exploration is this: to open our hearts, minds, and bodies to the journey – the teachings of the people and the whisperings of the land – to take home with us more than pictures and tinkling souvenirs; to take home harmony.[45]

Sol Guide Method – Body

With Sol Guide Method you'll use physical movement to help your clients leave the stress of every day life behind and assist their minds to reach a focused, relaxed state. This helps your clients be present in their bodies, making it easier for a fun, personal connection with the outdoors to occur. It's this focused combination of body/mind/nature that helps the client feel rejuvenated and recharged by their experience.

You've probably experienced the personal chatter that often creeps into a workout in the gym or studio. Your clients will tell you about the grand kids, the annoying man at work, and what their dog ate for breakfast. The conversations can be fun and enhance our relationships, but they can also become a distraction. Use the change of venue in the outdoors to stay focused and enjoy a refreshing break from the day-to-day pressures of indoor training. Be prepared – Mother Nature is a wonderful equalizer. Experiences and conversations in the outdoors can reach a much more intimate level. This can be vulnerable, even scary territory for you and your client. Be careful to respect professional boundaries but don't be afraid to let your compassionate self shine through. Enjoy it!

The goal in leading an outdoor fitness retreat of any kind is not to record countless miles spinning or running while rocking out to your favorite music. You may very well use wearable fitness technology or an app to track miles and progress. The analytics and data are both informative and fun. Keep in mind that the goal is to break free from our modern day dependence on screens and create an experience where the body, mind, and nature combine into one harmonious chorus. This is how the human race used to exist on a day-to-day basis. Can you imagine?

You can start working into this type of exercise format today. Do these exercises and activities with your clients now, in your indoor training environment. Before you take it outside, find a green space nearby that will provide a quiet setting for the mindfulness part of the practice. Once you're ready to lead full-on fitness adventures in the outdoors you'll apply this same technique and flow with your natural surroundings.

Rather than be the person just giving directions, it's fun to perform the exercises with your client. When training more than one person or a small group, it's more comfortable to form a circle than it is for you to stand in front like the traditional group exercise class. You're all in this together, and for once you get to move with your clients too, instead of just telling them what to do all the time.

ACTIVITY

Standing in place, complete a series of the dynamic warm-up (you'll learn the dynamic exercise sequences later in the Body-Weight Exercise Arsenal chapter): high knees, butt kickers, and straight leg kicks.

Next, with feet hip-width apart, sink into 15 slow squats. Drop to the hands and hold a plank position for about 30 seconds to one minute. Return to standing and repeat the sequence, only this time perform the squats a little faster. When you drop into plank, widen the legs or do a set of mountain climbers. Bear crawl your way across the floor to the center of the circle where you all come together. Balancing on one hand, reach up to give your neighbor a high five. Remaining in a plank position, walk or inch-worm your way back to the outskirts of the circle. Repeat this sequence two to three times, with each set becoming increasingly more challenging. Spend 15–20 minutes on this part of the workout.

Next, walk or lightly jog your way to a nearby green space, water's edge, orchard or field. Invite your client to set an intention of what they want to get out of this session today. Share with them the Navajo Beauty Way, the Blue Marble Game, or your own method of connecting to the outdoors.

Dedicate the session to something beautiful, a harmonious connection between mind, body, and nature. It's ideal if this walk/jog can take 10–20 minutes.

Notice how your client's energy should have quieted some. In this quiet space, settle into a series of breathing exercises. Start with 5-10 ribcage openers and encourage the clients to imagine breathing into all spaces of their lungs—into the lower back, the sides of the ribs, the diaphragm, even up under the collar bones. Do 10 each of the cleansing and energizing breaths. Vary the breathing exercises by doubling the time it takes to exhale. On the last breath of each set, encourage your client to take the biggest breath ever. Hold the breath after the inhalation as long as possible. Exhale, slowly. Spend 10-15 minutes breathing, depending on the stress level of your client.

Now, give your client 5-10 minutes of alone time in nature. Encourage them to find a place to sit quietly. If your client is an analytical person you can encourage them to use their five senses to observe their surroundings. What do they smell, touch, see, hear, and taste? If the person is more intuitive or deeply interested in nature and the universe, encourage them to listen to the messages nature might have for them. What does their intuition tell them?

End the quiet meditation time by walking or slowly jogging back to the starting point. Share any of your own observations and feelings. You can invite the client to share what they discovered during their journey too. You just might learn something new!

Reflection

It helps to reflect back to people what you see in them. I often work with business travelers to Utah. They arrive looking haggard and tense. After a few hours of exercising and playing they're laughing, smiling, and literally appearing much younger. I still think that living an active life is the greatest anti-aging strategy!

JOURNAL ENTRY - MIND/BODY CONNECTION

Take some time to think about a mantra you could use to guide your clients to focus and enhance their mind/body connection. Use this exercise as an opportunity to brainstorm ways to help your clients stay engaged.

> **Example:** *Encourage your client to focus on their breathing. If possible, inhale through the nostrils and out the mouth. With each inhalation, imagine breathing in light and happiness. With each exhale, release all fears, doubts, and worries. Inhale health. Inhale love, joy, and pleasure. Exhale pain, disappointment, and grief. Allow enough time for 5 – 10 of these breaths. Keep the feet hip-width apart and the knees soft, the shoulders relaxed. The eyes can be open or closed. Remind them as you move to "check in with the mind, check in with the body, check in with the emotions, and smile. Feel harmony in your mind, your body, and your emotions. Smile."*

Sol Guide Method – Mind

Think about the number of hours people all over the world spend mindlessly cranking out minutes on an elliptical machine each day. Sure, maybe they are listening to music or thinking about their meetings later in the day. They are not present in the moment, inside their own bodies. It's easy to ignore the mental fitness component of exercise while working out on traditional gym cardio equipment. My point isn't to dismiss doing cardio in the gym, rather I want to emphasize that a healthy body is incomplete without a healthy mind.

The mindfulness component of Sol Guide Method deliberately follows and builds on the foundation of physical exercise. First the body was used to generate blood flow, warm up the muscles, and get the client's full attention. Now is the time to increase oxygen intake, focus the mind, and guide the client in the process of looking inward. Some people think that the word 'mindfulness' is loaded and intimidating; it really just refers to the state of simply being completely present and in the moment. Mindfulness practices can take many shapes and forms. You can set intentions, chant mantras, guide meditations and visualizations or lead scientific observations. Feel free to use the method that feels right for the setting and your client in that moment.

IMPORTANT!

It's common for the mindfulness exercises to take a spiritual turn; but it's up to you to select the practice that matches the goals and objectives of your client. Mindfulness work is a time to be aware of the diversity of backgrounds and beliefs in the world. Most of the time, in a professional setting, your choice of words will be universal and free from dogma. If you're working with a particular sect or church group in your community it may be appropriate to refer to deity using specific names and terms. You may choose to steer clear of spiritual references altogether, using only scientific terms or descriptions of the exercise. The key is to be respectful of the demographic and situation you are working in.

This is a fantastic window to take advantage of the brief moments you and your clients have to be unplugged and outdoors in a spectacular natural setting! Approach this work with a pure intent. Assist the client to reach a relaxed state of mind—and prepare for the magic to unfold.

Meditation

What are the benefits of meditation? Similar to being in the outdoors, the body reaps extensive psychological and physiological benefits from meditation. These benefits include decreased anxiety and depression, decreased irritability, improved learning ability and memory, lowered levels of the stress hormone cortisol, deeper sleep patterns, and increased oxygen uptake.

ACTIVITY

Walking Meditation

Here's a very simple walking meditation for you to try today. The goal is to simply be 100% present with this activity. Whenever you catch your mind wandering, gently bring it back to the walking and begin again. It's helpful to have a beginning and end destination in mind when you do this, like walking from the bottom of the hill to the top, for example.

Step 1. Count the number of steps it takes for you to take one relaxed inhale. Say you take four steps while you inhale.

Step 2. As you exhale, double the number of steps of your inhale, so make your exhale last eight steps.

Step 3. Continue walking and breathing in this pattern and watch how the numbers change. Eventually you'll settle into a consistent number of inhales and exhales that matches your pace. What are your numbers?

Matching

Circle the correct term(s) regarding the benefits of mindfulness. Not all terms will be used.

Mindfulness has what kind of effect on the following emotions?

1. Anxiety and depression
        decreased or increased

2. Irritability
        decreased or increased

3. Learning ability and memory
        improved or decreased

4. Levels of cortisol, the stress hormone
        lowered or increased

5. Sleep patterns
        deeper or less deep

6. Air flow to the lungs
        increased or decreased

Mindfulness - Intention Setting

I want to introduce the idea of setting an intention with a quick personal story.

MEL SAYS

In 2009 I guided a fitness adventure for three clients on a 3-day Inca Trail Trek to Machu Picchu, Peru. Our first stop was Cusco, elevation 12,000 feet. There are horror stories of tourists sidelined by skull-splitting headaches in Cusco, so I spent the summer training and living at high elevations in Colorado and Utah. I arrived in Cusco a few days before my clients did, just in case I had bad luck and got altitude sickness.

Luckily the altitude didn't bother me. The cobblestone streets led me around town and eventually to a shaman who taught private yoga lessons. Grateful for an hour of self-care before my clients arrived, I had one of the best yoga sessions I've ever had. Before any instruction began, the teacher invited me to be open and receptive to what this magical land of the ancient Inca had to offer me. The intention stuck with me. Through the unexpected ups and downs of the next week traveling Peru with my clients, I was able to see what I had to learn.

I've used this same intention many times to welcome clients on their fitness adventures. Trust me – while your client thinks all they want to do is cross a bucket list adventure off their list, there is always an underlying yearning just waiting to be fulfilled. Taking a moment to help your client connect with their intention can help turn that yearning into a reality.

Just what is intention and why use it? Intention is the mindset you bring to an action— what you want to deliberately achieve. A good example of using intention is performing a training run with a goal in mind. Maybe you time a set distance and compare it to last week's times. You could visualize your performance by imagining breathing at a slow and even pace, arms relaxed at your sides, legs moving effortlessly across the land. An example of the opposite of intent is mindlessly running on the treadmill while reading a novel or texting a friend.

Research has shown one of the best ways to help clients reduce stress is to help them focus on the task at hand. In other words, help them to be present. Once the mind and body connect through intentional action, anything is possible. Remember, this is where the 'flow' state can be reached. You may know what that feels like. Can you imagine guiding someone into that feeling for the first time? It's an incredibly rewarding experience!

Bringing intention to action yields powerful, proven results.

EXAMPLE

Say you're about to hike in Topanga State Park outside of L.A. with a group of five young professionals on a Saturday morning. Here's how to set an intention for the day:

Welcome to fitness adventures with [the name of your business]! We're about to give your mind and body it's daily dose of nature cure. Topanga State Park is a rugged, steep and scenic escape from the city. Long before L.A. was built, the Chumash Indians called these mountains home, and it was a critical source of food and resources. Before we start working out, I'd like to invite you to set an intention to receive the rejuvenating and grounding influence the mountain offers you. Take just a minute to connect with the desire that brought you here this morning. Power it up and bring it to the forefront of your mind as we move, and watch what happens.

What kind of intention can you invite your clients to use? Brainstorm examples here.

What's your intention for wellness today?

What kind of movement will you do that causes your intention to come to fruition?

What types of food will you eat to wake up your taste buds and delight your senses?

How does it feel to bring the power of intentional thought to your everyday workout?

Mindfulness - Navajo Beauty Way

The Navajo, or Diné, are a band of American Indians who occupy a large reservation on the Colorado Plateau landscape in Arizona. Growing up in Utah, I had Navajo friends who danced at my birthday parties. The way the bells and feathers of their costumes moved to the rhythm of their dances mesmerized me. Later, when I lived on the Utah/ Arizona border, Navajo friends shared their culture with me in ways that I've learned to incorporate into my work as a guide. What are the tribes near you and how can you learn from their native rituals?

Hózhó Ná asha dó

An essential facet of Navajo life is Hózho, which means balance and harmony.[46] Many English concepts are included in Hózho, including beauty, perfection, harmony, success, goodness, normality, well being, blessedness, and happiness.

During a Navajo Beauty Way ceremony, the patient (the person who is ill) is seeking to re-establish balance and beauty in her life.

There are endless reasons we lose balance and harmony in our lives. A few examples include:

- illness
- day-to-day pressure
- being plugged in all the time
- grief
- trauma
- politics

To the Navajo there is only one cure for every day ailments. One must find the way to beauty, and if one wanders away from this way, from the Beauty Way, then one must re-establish one's link to the natural world in order to regain it.

To *Walk in Beauty* means not only walking physically. Primarily it means being in harmony with all things and all people, with all objects, animals, feelings, plants, weather and all the events in your life. It means being at peace, serene in the knowledge that all around you is well and that you are well with everything in your life. You accept and are accepted. There is nothing that pulls you in one direction or the other. The polarities are neutralized and you are one with everything.

MEL SAYS

I've hiked on both coasts of the U.S. and on five continents. Hiking is a fantastic way to explore the countryside and see indigenous people and cultures. Imagine hiking through a bamboo forest in Bali, Indonesia. You can hear music playing nearby, but the vines and trees are so thick all you can see is the occasional backside of the family cow. A sinewy, tanned man wearing a loincloth swings his scythe while submerged above his ankles in wet rice paddies. A native woman washes her clothes in an irrigation ditch as her two little boys play nearby.

What have you experienced during your wanderings?

I like to share the Beauty Way Ceremony with clients before leading them on a hike in the desert or the mountains. The ceremony addresses our basic human need for balanced harmony in a very non-threatening way. You'll experience the ceremony on the next page. You are welcome to follow along with the words, but I recommend you also listen to it in a quiet place with your eyes closed. Try being intentionally mindful. Does this concept resonate with you?

Walk in Beauty

You are ready to <u>Walk in Beauty.</u>

ACTIVITY

In beauty may I walk
All day long may I walk
Through the returning seasons may I walk
Beautifully I will possess again
Beautifully birds
Beautifully joyful birds
On the trail marked with pollen may I walk
With grasshoppers about my feet may I walk
With dew about my feet may I walk
With beauty may I walk
With beauty before me may I walk
With beauty behind me may I walk
With beauty above me may I walk
With beauty above me may I walk
Today I will walk out, today everything negative will leave me
I will be as I was before
I will have a cool breeze over my body
I will have a light body
I will be happy forever
Nothing will hinder me
In old age, wandering on a trail of beauty, lively, may I walk
In old age, wandering on a trail of beauty, living again, may I walk
It is finished in beauty
It is finished in beauty[47]

JOURNAL ENTRY – A WALK IN BEAUTY

A Walk in Beauty is a powerful tool to help your clients be mindful, to form their own connection with Mother Nature, and to gain understanding of a different culture.

How can you use this ceremony with your own clients?

Sol Guide - Nature

Sol Guide Method is to be applied to pure outdoor experiences. By that I mean getting out of the city. Unless you live in Alaska with acres of wilderness out your front door, you will actually need to take a mini-trip somewhere. You could travel 15 minutes or 2 hours, depending on your goal. Your retreat can last a few hours, a half-day, a full day, or even multiple-days. For multi-day adventures, you'll need some advanced training.

You may ask, "Can I lead the nature component of Sol Guide Method in a city park?" That's a good question.

The answer is yes, you certainly can, but don't mistake this program for a boot camp. A real fitness retreat offers your clients so much more than a booty-busting sweat session at the park. This is your chance to introduce your clients to a lifestyle of activity that they'll enjoy for the rest of their life. It's not about creating dependence on you as their instructor. Rather, it's about helping your clients reconnect with that innate state of human motion. Think of the impact one event could have on their health and happiness!

Still not clear why this isn't a boot camp? Well, believe it or not, researchers distinguish between physical activity and physical exercise. Physical activity is defined as, "any bodily movement produced by skeletal muscles that requires energy expenditure." Physical exercise is, "a subcategory of physical activity that is planned, structured, repetitive, and purposeful in the sense that the improvement or maintenance of one or more components of physical fitness is the objective."[48]

There's a very fine line separating these two types of movements, especially when you factor a teacher or guide is giving instructions, like you do in your current practice and will continue to do as you implement Sol Guide Method principles. Can you see the difference between going for a hike to a spectacular waterfall or kayaking under the Aurora Borealis and doing a bunch of burpees at the elementary school playground? We're talking about completely different paradigms, even when you add the instructional warm up and cool down.

Reading this course and studying the Sol Guide Method does not automatically qualify you to take your clients on a rock-climbing trip, even if you're a recreational climber. Unless you have the proper licensing, credentials, insurance and permits, don't even think about it. Instead, take a six-week course and get certified. Or, even easier, partner with a professional climbing company to lead the trip for you under their permits and insurance.

> **IMPORTANT!**
>
> I explore the legal and business aspects of guiding outdoor fitness retreats in great detail in *Adventure's in MOTHER NATURE'S GYM The Business Workbook*. If you're serious about implementing the principles taught in this course into your own outdoor fitness retreat, you'll want to pick up *The Business Workbook*. Including detailed planning methods, sample safety talks, and gear lists, *The Business Workbook* will walk you step by step through the practical steps of setting up your operation and keeping clients safe in the outdoors.

What is Nature?

If nature isn't found on the playground, where is it? There are endless sources describing nature, but the one that resonates most closely with Sol Guide Method is described by author Richard Louv in his book on nature-deficit disorder:

> Natural wildness: biodiversity, abundance…nature is reflected in our capacity for wonder. Nasci. To be born. Though we often see ourselves as separate from nature, humans are also part of that wildness.[49]

In his powerful book Scattered, Gabor Maté says, "the parent who never takes his child out into nature, away from the city, is depriving him not only of wonderful experiences but also of a powerfully harmonizing influence for the mind. There is matchless unity, harmony and peace in nature—all that is lacking, in other words, in the ADD mind."[50]

The way Sol Guide Method utilizes nature is grounded in theories of Recreation Management. "Outdoor recreation in particular—think hiking, rafting, surfing, skiing, camping—takes place in an environment that has naturally occurring challenges and consequences." Challenges you may face "out there" include falling off the paddleboard or skiing in a big snowstorm. The rewards of overcoming these challenges include "teaching persistence and building confidence."[51]

Nature - The Setting

Several factors that will dictate your chosen outdoor setting include:

- client goals
- location
- weather
- budget
- time constraints

Keep in mind the way the environment specifically supports the mind and body as you plan your fitness retreat (remember the blue mind, green mind, and red mind concepts in Part Three).

You've laid the foundation that prepares your client to be fully engaged in the outdoors: muscles and joint stabilizers are fired; the mind is focused, alert, and present; cascades of neurotransmitters and feel-good hormones have begun to create a feeling of happiness. Now you're ready to apply the sport-specific component of the Sol Guide Method.

Use the exercise sequences in the Body-Weight Exercise Arsenal (Part Six) and mindfulness exercises as warm ups or cool downs and then pair them with countless outdoor activities. My specialties as a guide are hiking, cycling, and stand up paddling. There are endless possibilities, including water-based activities like surfing, kayaking, or open-water swimming. Land-based activities like canyoneering, rock-climbing, and trekking take the adrenaline factor to the next level, as does mountain biking on single track.

JOURNAL ENTRY – NATURE ADVENTURE SETTINGS

Natural settings for a half-day or full-day fitness adventure are not likely to be too far from your location. Take the time to find the real gems near your home, even if you live in an urban area.

Do some research and find four nearby locations that would be ideal for a half-day or full-day fitness retreat. Ust this journal entry to name each of the four places and their locations, as well as outlining the considerations on the following page.

Journal Entry, continued…

1. Distance and time to travel to the location
2. Ideal outdoor recreation and body-weight exercises to do
3. Unique historical/cultural/natural resources things to see and do
4. Costs, permits required, agency or company contact person

Need some hints on where to start your research? Try researching the State and Federal Government resources found at the links listed below:

America's State Parks at americasstateparks.org/
National Park Conservation Association at npca.org/
National Wildlife Federation at nwf.org/naturefind.aspx
Discover the Forest at discovertheforest.org/
ParkRx at parkrx.org

Bridging the Gap - Fitness Meets Adventure

The word fitness conjures images of busy gyms, smelly yoga studios, and racks of free weights for many of us. Sol Guide Method requires a paradigm shift in the way mind/body professionals approach fitness. With Sol Guide Method, *fitness is more than a gym workout – it's a way of life!*

Sol Guide Method will empower you as you introduce a new lifestyle to your clients. The outdoor activities will draw you and your client closer to the land and the natural rhythms of our ancestors as you bridge the gap between two modern day industries, outdoor and wellness. Traditional gyms and spas occupy a tidy indoor niche, while the outdoor industry occupies their expansive outdoor space. With outdoor fitness retreats you will successfully mix and blend the two.

You need a basic understanding of who the players in the outdoor space are in order to understand how to expertly bridge the gap between the two industries. Knowing what options your clients have for fulfilling their adventure-seeking and/or healthy vacation desires will give you an edge as you carve out your own unique positioning in the market.

Spa

Your clients have most likely visited a destination spa, where they can exercise all day every day, eat nutritious food, and get some pampering. The spa employs trainers and every kind of group exercise instructor imaginable. Destination spa instructors perform services for people day in and day out. They may form a personal connection with the guests, but more than likely these connections are fleeting.

There's a time and place for everything, and if your clients are anything like mine, at some point they'll grow tired of the destination spa routine and off-the-rack adventure trips. They'll want to see their training program applied to a real world setting. Your clients may be hungry for an experience that will edify and transform them. They'll want to go on an adventure with you because they trust you and know that you care about them.

Outfitters and Tour Operators

Most outdoor guide companies (in the adventure travel and outdoor industries these companies are called outfitters and guides or tour operators) operate the same trip each day. They might specialize in white water rafting trips on a particular stretch of river in Veracruz, Mexico, or guiding via ferratas on the Utah / Arizona border. There are tour operators all over the world and particularly in Europe, who specialize in high-end cycling trips through their favorite wine country in Provence, France or Prague in the Czech Republic, for example.

Outfitters and guides and tour operations function completely different from the fitness industry. Rarely do they have the training in anatomy or exercise science that mind/ body professionals have. Rather than tailor a trip to the client's physical abilities, most of the time the clients must custom-fit themselves to the trip. It's like shopping for a wedding dress – you can buy a pretty dress off the rack much cheaper than you can have the perfect fit custom designed.

Chances are clients in every price range have paid for a guided outdoor experience doing some form of activity. Common active vacations include cycling and hiking tours and safaris. Travelers may pay top dollar for a private trip or pay a little less to join a group adventure (without knowing what kind of people they'll meet).

The ability to create custom fitness adventures is what makes you so unique! Do you realize what you have to offer the outdoor, travel, destination spa and wellness industries? Your chance of leading a successful outdoor fitness adventure skyrockets when you can assess the client's physical fitness—or lack thereof—and create an experience just for them. Rather than drive your client hard all day on a grueling hike, you'll pick the right distance, time, and terrain to highlight your client's physical capacity.

Via Ferrata – Known as the Iron Road, via ferrata's were originally built in the Dolomite mountain range in Italy during World War I. The Italian army used them to gain direct access to their enemies rather than travel around the entire range. Via ferrata's are appearing in North America in Utah and Colorado. They're a great way to get first-time climbers out on the rock or weaker climbers to the top of an epic cliff with less strain.

Tour Operator – A tour operator is a company within the travel industry that specializes in packaging and selling an all-inclusive trip or itinerary. The trip price may include flights and transportation, hotels, restaurants, as well as costs for all guide and entertainment services while on location.

Outfitter and Guide – An outfitter and guide is a company that specializes in a type of guided outdoor activity, typically in a specific location. Many states use this designation as a business license that must be registered. For example, in the State of Utah my business Sol Fitness Adventures needs to be registered as an outfitter and guide when I guide stand up paddling fitness retreats at Glen Canyon National Recreation Area (also known as Lake Powell). Types of business operations that may qualify as outfitters and guides include hunting guides, Jeep tours, river companies, rock climbing guides, rope courses, stand up paddle and kayaking guides, mountain biking tours. If you're about to lead a commercial trip that includes one of these activities, that could include you.

I'll walk you through the process of designing an outdoor fitness adventure in Part Five, Creating Outdoor Fitness Retreats. You'll learn how to do everything from client assessment to designing a retreat that delivers targeted results.

Putting it all Together

I've presented the three main facets of Sol Guide Method – body, mind, and nature - at a high level thus far. Now I want to present you with some snapshots of what a fitness adventure may look like as you implement this method. Remember, this program does not give you specific recipes to follow because your own fitness adventures will be highly customized. You'll learn more about fitness adventure program design in Part Five.

For now, let's break down the planning stages of a sample-hiking trip. Imagine yourself creating a hiking trip to Maine for a group of clients and try to anticipate what aspects you will need to plan in order to make it a success. The questions that follow are meant to, 1) help you understand the scope of what it takes to create a retreat, 2) let you figure out your own method of researching and planning trip details, 3) reveal that there may not be one right answer, and 4) help you think of retreat locations near your own home.

A Maine Hiking Trip - A Scenario

Five women who play tennis together approach you to take them on an outdoor fitness trip. They're close friends in their late 40's. They appear to be in good shape and all belong to the local gym, where they work out together and provide a solid support group for one another. They want to go on a hike that will give them enough elevation to challenge their fitness levels and get them out into nature. They're very busy and some have children at home so it's necessary for the entire outing, including travel time, to fit into one day, ideally less than 10-hours door to door.

You, along with the clients, live in Maine. After some research, you realize that White Cap Mountain, located on the Appalachian Trail, is only a 45-minute drive away. You can start and end the hike at the Sidney Tappan Campsite, which has a nice field for warming up and cooling down.

Your Turn – Research the Logistics

    1. How far is the hike from Sidney Tappan Campsite to the peak of White Cap?
    2. Can the hike be done in a day?

3. Would the hike suit your clients objectives and be a good match for their fitness levels?

4. What elevation is White Cap at the peak?

5. How will you get there?

Your Turn – Anticipate Client Needs

1. What will you do for food and drinks?

2. What if your client is an Instagram influencer and needs to post content along the way?

3. Where are the bathrooms and what will you do if someone has never gone in the woods?

4. What's the weather prediction?

5. What kind of personal gear is necessary for the hike?

Your Turn – Pre-Trip Preparations

1. When are you going to make a site visit and run through the trip on your own?

2. What are the must-see sights along the drive and trail?

3. What kind of native plants and animals can you expect to see and how will you help your clients identify them?

4. Is there any historical significance to the area?

5. What is the geologic history of the mountain?

Your Turn – Designing the Body and Mind Components

Nothing feels worse than being on a hike and charging full speed from the very first step. In fact, this can cause a dangerous shock to the heart resulting in tachycardia. To warm up for the hike, you will want to spend at least 15-minutes on a flat surface at the campsite, moving all the large muscle groups to increase blood flow and slowly preparing the heart for an increased workload.

1. Knowing the distance of your hike, what will you do for warm up exercises?

2. What exercises will combine to make a good cool down regimen after the hike?

3. How will you manage doing a workout on dirt or grass?

4. What can you do to help the clients remain present throughout the day?

5. What special talents do you have that can shine in this setting that you aren't able to utilize in a gym setting?

Review - Sol Guide Method

Matching

Match the term to the appropriate space. Not all terms will be used.

1. The primary goal of Sol Guide Method is to accomplish the following:

engage   a._____ the body
surround   b. _____ the spirits
change   c. _____ the senses in nature
lift
strengthen
challenge

Multiple Choice

Select the answer that best fits the statement.

1.   The Sol Guide Method approach to fitness is a _____.

   a. Specifically outlined regimen
   b. Complicated sequence of activities
   c. Way of life
   d. Closely guarded secret

2.   The mindset you bring to an action, what you want to deliberately achieve.

   a. Mindfulness
   b. Flow
   c. Intention
   d. Wellness

3.   Flow is achieved when you are doing which two important things simultaneously (select both terms)?

   a. Arousal
   b. Being mindful
   c. Control
   d. Exercising

4.   Which of the following is not one of the three important ideas upon which Sol Guide Method is founded?

   a. Body
   b. Nature
   c. Mind
   d. Oxygen

5.   The state of simply being completely present and in the moment.

   a. Mindfulness

b. Joy

c. Exhaustion

d. Intentional

6. The state of being fit.

a. Wellness

b. Health

c. Peace

d. Fitness

7. Sol Guide Method uses _____ to facilitate a fit mind and a fit body.

a. Specific exercise sequences

b. Natural settings

c. Diet and exercise

d. Weights and exercise machines

8. The best time to invite clients to set an intention is _____.

a. At the beginning of the session

b. At least 24 hours before the session

c. After the session

d. During the session

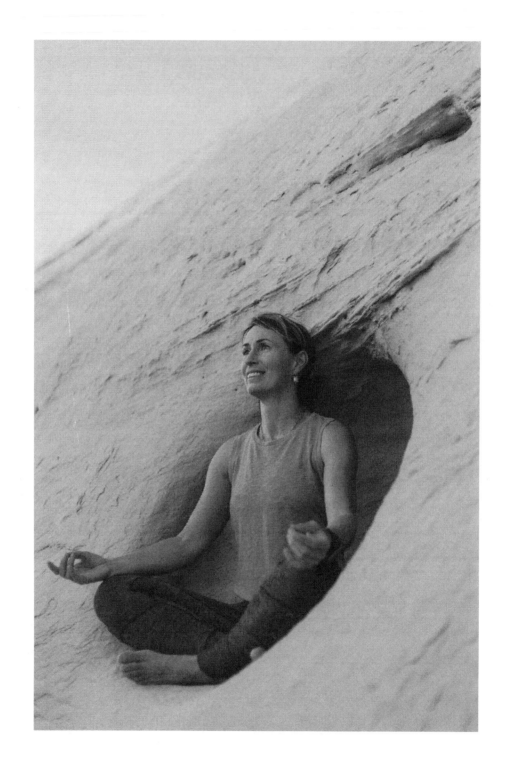

ADVENTURES IN MOTHER NATURE'S GYM

PART FOUR
THE OUTDOOR FITNESS GUIDE

"Be grateful for whoever comes, because each guest

has been sent as a guide from beyond." - RUMI

What is a Guide?

Years ago, educational philosophy underwent a major shift. Some declared that the role of teachers should not be "the sage on the stage" who hands out information and gives commands. The teacher, instead, should be, "the guide on the side" who allows the student to learn, grow, and even teach others, all while helping, answering questions and offering assistance.

Sol Guide Method subscribes to this theory as well. The personality of an all-knowing yoga guru or a bombastic boot-camp instructor won't work during an outdoor fitness retreat. People embark on a retreat seeking something they can't get out of the everyday group exercise class or personal training session. For some it's the desire to see the fitness levels they've developed through their indoor training program applied to a real-world setting. For others a retreat represents a vacation that requires the sacrifice of time and money to spend time with family or try something new – and with that sacrifice comes great expectations.

Sol Guide Method will help you become a guide. That's a loaded word. When a guide says "come, follow me," he's not giving a command; he's extending an invitation. Good guides don't lead by force or coercion, through ego or intimidation. A true leader shows his followers the way through strong and confident action.

You want your clients to follow you into those outdoor places that may scare and challenge them—places that they know they cannot, or will not, go without you. First you have to demonstrate that you're worthy of their trust and respect. How do you do that? First you have to earn that trust and respect.

Guide Traits

There are many words that describe a guide. Way-shower, leader, teacher, exemplar, shepherd, and instructor are all terms that come to mind. To be a great guide requires character traits like confidence, integrity, dignity, compassion, fortitude, kindness, boldness, bravery, selflessness, patience, precision, strength, skill, and intuition.

Most professionals in the fitness and mind/body industries inherently possess or have developed many of the qualities required of a guide. Making the transition to guiding clients in the outdoors is a natural progression that simply requires developing the competence to work in that new arena. As with any endeavor, becoming the expert takes time and dedication.

A great guide also has to be very self-aware. On one hand, you must have complete confidence in yourself. You trust your ability and know you're prepared. You could even go as far as to say you're a "badass."

You need to be humble enough to know your own limits and to adapt to the situation, like bad weather or struggling clients. You may be able to reach the mountain peak you've dreamed of summiting within a certain time; but your clients may not make it before the dark storm lurking on the horizon rolls in. What are you going to do: honor your client's pace by turning back or push them beyond their limits and put them in a dangerous situation?

MEL SAYS

I've been privileged to work with many great guides, both in the outdoors and in the fitness studio. Those who I partner with to run my trips in southern Utah work in extremely remote and challenging conditions on a regular basis. They can smell rain on the wind, even when there isn't a cloud in the sky directly overhead. These aren't the adventure travel guides who dress for dinner and sip fine wine with clients in Provence, France (not that I wouldn't if given the opportunity!). These are the specialists you want to seek out and partner with when the stakes are high and safety and expertise are paramount.

Guide Limitations

I learned the "know your limits and learn to adapt" lesson the hard way once. Luckily I was by myself and not leading any clients the day I decided to take on Mother Nature and act like an arrogant outdoorswoman. Although I had witnessed several flash floods and knew the signs to watch for, there was a day when I exercised extremely poor judgment while hiking in a slot canyon in southern Utah. I was so fixated on my destination that, in spite of clear signs that I was in danger, I refused to turn around and hike out.

Below is an excerpt from my short story "Slot Canyon Body Slam," published in *CARSON Magazine*:

"As I huddled under the safety of an enormous overhanging wall, drank some water, and took a few deep breaths, I considered the seriousness of the situation. It was already raining hard, I still had more than four miles to go to reach the exit, and even if the pending flash flood wasn't deadly, I could still easily be trapped here overnight. In no mood to spend the night in the canyon, I mixed a high calorie energy drink, took a few bites of a granola bar, and continued down the slippery slope to the creek. The wisdom of a fellow canyoneer guide rang in my ears, "when 100% of the 20% prediction of rain falls in your particular drainage, you do what you have to do to survive."[52]

That day taught me one of the most profound lessons in my life. In addition to grappling with the results of my poor decision-making I came face to face with my own mortality. There was a period of time during the ordeal that I *knew* I was going to die. My number was up; I was on my way to meet my Creator.

In a stroke of luck—or perhaps divine timing—I managed to outrun the flash flood and reach the exit route to safety with about five minutes to spare. There is, of course, much more to this story than what I've shared here, including a depth of spiritual insight that I feel has made me a much better person. It was only after I realized that I wasn't afraid to die that I decided I wasn't going to be afraid to really *live*.

It's certainly not necessary to survive a near death experience in order to be a great guide! It's that life energy I try to share with my clients when I'm 'out there' with them; many of whom are metaphorically and spiritually dying under the burdens of life and stress. I encourage you to draw from the lessons of the rich tapestry of your own life as you approach this work. Be prepared to share from your heart and soul, because while the fun of an outdoor fitness retreat may be what caught your clients attention, it's your ability to give them an encounter with life and Mother Nature that will transform their own lives.

JOURNAL ENTRY - KNOW YOUR LIMITS

Have you been in a situation either as a guide or as an adventurer where you were in over your head?
What was the situation?
How did you deal with it?
Write what you learned from that experience, and think about what you have to offer because of it.

The Role of a Guide

The varied responsibilities of a guide may feel new and intimidating when you first begin to implement the principles of Sol Guide Method. Though we fitness pros continue to learn new research and apply new techniques to help clients progress, we essentially repeat the same act every day, in the same space as the day before. The role of a guide takes on more responsibility than a one-hour indoor exercise session; it is very multi-dimensional. In comparison, the role of a traditional fitness instructor can be quite one-dimensional. This is probably the biggest reason why, once I began leading fitness retreats, there was no going back to full time personal training in the gym.

Unlike what the adventure travel industry at large would tell you, your role as a guide is much more than merely planning logistics or playing chauffeur. Your opportunity is to help others find their own hidden talents and strengths. Your job is to safely lead them through an experience that has the potential to transform. The duties related to gear, time, and travel are necessary, but your most important work is to lead others to a reconnection between themselves and the outdoors.

In certain situations, such as in the backcountry far from civilization, you literally *are* the lifeline to your clients, responsible to safely lead them in and out of remote venues. On other occasions you may have the luxury of hiring a local expert and allowing them to bear the weight of protecting and caring for all of you. In this case, you play the roll of "strong second" by assisting the lead guide to look after the comfort and safety of your clients.

IMPORTANT!

Assist your clients as they transfer skills mastered in the gym to physical challenges in an unfamiliar outdoor environment. Help others reach a new level of self-realization.

Remember this guide motto:

Lead. Assist. Help.

Fill in the Blank

Select the word from the list below that best matches the blank to complete the paragraph. Not all words will be used.

Help others find their own hidden _____ and strengths by safely _____ them into new territory. Lead others back to themselves, _____ them meet physical _____ in an unfamiliar outdoor _____ to reach a new level of self- _____ .

environment
spirituality
realization
talents

direct
challenges
leading
help
ailments

Guide Responsibilities

variety of outdoor fitness retreats and diversity of clients you can work with means it's likely that no two adventures will be exactly the same. That means you will need to adapt and be flexible. However, there are some basic responsibilities that are consistent, regardless of the adventure. Whether the fitness retreat will last for a few hours, a day, or multiple days, an outdoor fitness guide must become and expert at the following skill sets:

Logistics

Logistics are the nitty-gritty details, the small parts that make up the whole. If you want your outdoor fitness retreat to run like a well-oiled machine and feel and look seamless to your guests, the elements to hone in on include:

- Start and end times
- Start and end locations
- Trail markers
- Obstacles and route condition
- Total distance and mileage covered
- Locations for picnics or van support stops
- Address and directions to the nearest hospital
- Cell phone service
- Gas stations and restaurants
- Preparation of route notes
- Emergency contact numbers
- Prominent landmarks

Interpretation

As an outdoor fitness guide you do not need to know every type of plant or in-depth details of the geology of an area, but memorizing a few important facts to help your guests understand what makes a place unique will add value to the experience. Start by asking yourself the following questions:

- What makes its people and culture unique?

- What unique geological formations can you point out?
- How old is the earth in this location?
- How were the mountains formed? By earthquake or erosion?
- What about the water – is it man-made or natural?
- What pressures does the land face due to human population growth, political arguments, climate change, etc.?

Gear List and Inspection

You must make a complete inventory of all equipment, gear, and clothing required to make the retreat a success. In addition you'll need to provide clients with a complete gear list well in advance. If you can, and especially if the trip is multi-day and requires travel, do a gear inspection with your clients before the trip to make sure they are properly prepared. When renting bikes, stand up paddle boards, kayaks or other equipment from a supplier, perform a proper inspection with an employee of the shop present. Look for any type of "red flag" such as damage, loose or missing parts, or failure to require clients to sign a waiver.

Local Conditions

Remember to check the weather, road, water, and trail conditions well ahead of time. Be prepared to make last minute changes if necessary in order to keep the group safe. Reserve the right to change plans if conditions demand—and don't be afraid to do it.

Flexibility

Similar to training in the gym, conditions and people are in constant flux. Be prepared to adapt to existing and unexpected conditions as well as your clients varying energy levels, skill sets and abilities. Even after you have meticulously planned and prepared for every detail you must be able to change course if the situation requires it.

I go into great detail on these topics in *Adventures in MOTHER NATURE'S GYM The Business Manual* and recommend that you pick it up if you're serious about creating your own outdoor fitness retreats. It makes the perfect compliment to this book and will walk you step-by-step through the process of planning and monetizing your own trips.

Review – The Outdoor Fitness Guide

True or False

Select the answer that best fits the statement by circling true or false.

1. It is imperative to know every type of plant of an area where you will be guiding clients.

   True
   False

2. It is the client's responsibility to bring and maintain the equipment used on a retreat

   True
   False

3. It is a good idea for you, the guide, to have the contact information, address, and directions to the nearest hospital plugged into your phone or typed on a piece of paper.

   True
   False

4. It is a good idea for you, the guide, to have the contact information, address, and directions to the nearest hospital.

   True
   False

5. It is important to have options for even the most detailed adventure plan. Events and people are prone to unexpected circumstances.

   True
   False

6. Logistics refers to the legal ramifications and waivers that a client must sign before an adventure retreat.

   True
   False

Questions for the Self-Aware Guide

My objective in sharing Sol Guide Method is to teach how to lead clients on outdoor fitness retreats that are **transformational**, that help them reconnect to that ancient mindset of living powerfully and closely to earth energy. In essence, you are taking clients on a quest for wholeness. Similarly, by reading this course, you too are seeking something that can transform you personally and professionally. This, also, is a sort of quest.

What is a quest, anyway? *Merriam Webster's Dictionary* describes a quest as, "an act of looking carefully for someone or something." Related words include:

- Exploration
- Mission
- Pursuit
- Probe

I am going to ask you some probing details over the next several pages to help you define your quest as an outdoor fitness guide. Don't worry, you won't be graded and no one is going to read your answers! Take your time and work through these questions at your own pace.

JOURNAL ENTRY - WHAT'S IN IT FOR YOU?

No really, what do you want to get out of this course? Perhaps one of your passions is a particular outdoor sport and you want to find a way to share it with others and make a little money at the same time. Perhaps, in spite of your love for your clients, you're growing stale and getting bored of the monotony of indoor training.

Take a few minutes now to imagine the unlimited possibilities. Then, set your intention and write down specific goals related to your fitness practice and what you want it to grow into.

Sure, you could start describing all of the labels that describe you—a hipster or athlete, so-and-so's daughter, a personal trainer, a mystic, etc. All of those words may describe your style or what you do for a living, of course. What happens when you strip away the labels? Like the Cheshire Cat asked Alice in Wonderland: Who. Are. You? Don't just think about it - write it down.

Your Important Work

You may have heard that work ceases to be work when you enjoy it. What if you could take it a step further? What if work not only paid the bills but helped you and your clients feel whole and complete? If work is more than just fun and enjoyable, can it cease to be work and be a part of the bigger picture of growing and expanding as a human being?

Can you imagine what life looks like when you're engaged in doing the work you love?

Now, think about your broader pursuits in life. Maybe you dream of owning your own gym or studio. Perhaps leading an outdoor fitness retreat will help you expand your revenue streams and give your clients more ways to stay healthy. Or will it help you combine your passions and add variety to an otherwise stale work environment?

What does it look and feel like to be fully engaged in doing the work you love? Write it down.

Your Relationship to Your Own Body

Remember that one of the tenets of mindfulness is being present, both mentally and with the body. While I see this more in clients than in my fitness industry peers, some people spend so much time in their heads that they have virtually no connection to their body at all. As a young personal trainer I was so body-dominant that I'm not sure I was emotionally present and available much of the time. I've found that when I'm exercising outdoors, bringing the mind and the body into the present moment just seems to happen naturally.

The goal of an outdoor fitness retreat is to lead clients into a personal experience with nature through physical activity. It's essentially a process of self-discovery. To lead a successful retreat you will want your clients to feel challenged and focused, but not abused and defeated. Remember, this is what Csikszentmihaly referred to as 'flow state' (introduced in Part Three).

Many injuries could be avoided if people listened to their bodies rather than forcing it to achieve an unreasonable goal. A fitness retreat provides the opportunity to exercise the body and the mind, and you need the two to be in harmony to be successful. Much like a challenging indoor circuit or workout, you'll need to assist your clients to listen to their body and assess their abilities in order to respond to the challenges of the outdoors appropriately. You'll be more skilled at doing this if you develop this ability within yourself first.

How Do You Listen to Your Body?

The first step in listening to your body is to tell yourself that you will intentionally listen to your body and be mindful of it. Exercises in intention setting, mindfulness, and meditation allow you to connect to your body and help develop compassion. How can you have empathy and compassion for your clients if you refuse to have it for your own body?

Once you get into the workouts and guided outdoor activities, make sure you help your clients bring their minds back to the present consistently. As S.N. Goenka, a teacher of the Vipassana method taught, "the mind is a raging bull" that will run wild in a nearly hypnotic state where it can disconnect from the present moment completely (think about the times you have driven a car when your mind has wandered and you kind of "come back to yourself" ten blocks later).

Those of us in the mind/body professions have much to teach our clients about how to live with their bodies. We're kinesthetic beings, sometimes completely identified with what our athletic prowess and abilities can do. As a hard-driving athlete, developing compassion for my own body and learning to give myself permission to 'take rest' was very difficult for me. I took so much pleasure in pushing myself physically that it took me a long time to figure out how to be in balance and listen to my intuition. I shared my own journey of discovery with the ATHLETA community in an online essay called Mind, Body, and Spirit in Harmony:

"...I silenced my fears and insecurities behind a false sense of myself.

As long as my body looked and performed perfectly on the outside

I was in control, and scary events in life had no power over me.

If the scars on my scarecrow body could talk they would tell you a

different story: There's the three-inch incision near my left armpit that

marks a failed surgery to stop my shoulder from dislocating the three-

inch keloid [scar] on my left knee tells of the horrific night the doctor

told me I had nothing attaching my upper leg to the lower, and that

it might have to be amputated; the one-inch row of perfect stitches in

my left thigh reminds me of the firm warning I received from the ER

nurse that I would not compete in an adventure race that weekend; the

two-inch aged stitch above my right hip that no bikini can hide..."[53]

The story continues as I detail the rock-climbing incident that finally led me to seek balance by working on my inward life (my mental health). Judging from my own peer group and colleagues I suspect that many of you studying this course can relate in your own way to being body-dominant. I've always felt that the hardest part of healing from injury is dealing with the mental aspects. I also realize what an important role my own injuries and healing journey have played in my ability to successfully empathize, guide, and even love my own clients through their outdoor fitness retreats.

JOURNAL ENTRY – YOUR RELATIONSHIP TO YOUR OWN BODY

Who are you in relation to your body?
Are you comfortable in your own skin?
Have you ever been injured, lost a game or failed to reach a fitness goal?
What parts of your body hold you back from looking in the mirror every day and declaring how amazing you are?
Can you celebrate your body as the amazing gift that it is?

Mother Nature

I talk about the importance of nature throughout this program. What is nature? Nature isn't simply something that exists once you get far away from the city . . . nature is the earth upon which all of life is built. This earth was here long before us and will be here long after we are gone. When I stress the importance of connecting with nature, I want you to connect to the timeless earth.

For millennia, men, women and children lived their lives in harmony with the earth on which they lived. The rising and setting of the sun dictated daily activities. The ebb and flow of tides guided fishing and sailing routes. The coming and going of seasons brought bounty and famine. Humans were *of* the earth . . . not just *on* the earth.

It seems progress has inched us further and further from a meaningful and personal connection to the earth. We separate ourselves from the climate with efficient, cooled and heated homes. We separate ourselves from daily light cycles with electric lighting. We physically separate ourselves from one another with technology like cell phones and the Internet. And what is the price of this? What happens when we are disconnected from the very life-giving nature that we were once part of? Often it is our sense of wholeness and wellness that we sacrifice. We succumb to stress from the artificial world. We look to pills for sleep, happiness, and serenity.

What if we move backward, to our roots, and reconnect with the earth as we were meant to? We can regain our sense of self and place in this world and the wholeness that comes with knowing that we too are an important part of nature.

How Do You Reconnect with Mother Nature?

'Reconnecting to the earth' may sound completely woo-woo and corny to some, while others may have an inherent understanding of the role nature plays to their own well-being. For some of you urban dwellers to reconnect with the earth, you may need to take some time and intentionally submerse yourself in the things that you may have taken for granted for some time. If you just can't seem to find your way back, or have never experienced the joy and wonder of being outdoors – come and visit me in Utah, I'll help you!

Below are some of my favorite ways to reconnect with our blue planet, the entity many indigenous people know intimately as *Mother Earth*.

EXAMPLE

Get up early and watch a sunrise alone from a good vantage point.

Sit still at the edge of the surf as the tide comes in, allowing it to slowly envelops your toes, your knees, your hips.

Look up to the sky and try to find all the constellations you can **without** an app to help you.

Research what kind of local farms you can find near you, and if you can visit or help do some work.

Dig in the dirt. Most children love to play in the dirt – then we grow up and become afraid of it! Buy some native plants and get your hands dirty as you cultivate the soil in your yard or neighborhood community garden.

Get grounded. Find a nice patch of grass or swath of sand and walk or stand without shoes; sit in the grass; cross a stream. Allow your body to feel the Earth and your senses to take it all in.

Carry a special 'worry stone.' Find a small, round river stone and carry it in your pocket as a reminder of your connection to earth. When you feel stressed, rub your thumb across it, focusing on the touch.

Who are you in relation to this blue planet you call home?

Do you insist on eating organic or could you care less where your food comes from?

Does the idea of being "out there" in nature scare you a little, or excite and thrill you?

Did you ever pick up worms after a summer rain or play with frogs when you were little?

What's your ideal outdoor setting to play or relax in?

Do you have somewhere you can go, or is the closest outdoor location a far off and imaginary image on Instagram?

Client Relationships

For a guide to quickly connect with clients, it helps to take an interest in their lives. You need to know what's important to them, what they fear, and what they want to get out of attending your outdoor fitness retreat. Understanding your clients motivations is not a burden of being a guide - it is one of the many benefits.

Make sure you take the time to fully understand what your clients are asking of you and the relationship that is created in being their guide. They are putting a great amount of trust in you and are dependent upon you to:

- Guide them safely into and out of outdoor destinations
- Educate them about their natural surroundings
- Lead them through transformative mental and physical experiences
- Challenge while setting them up for success
- Teach them proper technique

Let's face it, that's a lot of pressure to put on a guide! You will be paid back for your devotion to your clients in more than just dollars and cents. As you guide people from different backgrounds, different regions, and different religions, you will learn new things every day. The bond forged through trust and care is a unique one, and is often more valuable than any photograph, bucket list accomplishment or bragging right gained on a particular adventure. Make sure you take the time to cherish and reflect on the value of this very special relationship you have cultivated with your clients. You did that!

In 2014 YourLifeIsATrip.com, the #1 Website for experiential Storytelling and Narrative Travel Writing, published an essay that I wrote called "Confessions of a Tour Guide." The story shared what went on in my mind when the pressure was on during one of my hiking trips to The Wave, an iconic and extremely remote landscape located on the Utah / Arizona border. The story is available in full online if you want to know all the juicy details, but for the purposes of this book I'll share just a few paragraphs that highlight what being a guide means to me.

   "What I learned that day was a metaphor for life as well: there are

   times when we can visualize where we want to go, but we don't know the way. Our path may be strewn with obstacles and setbacks or we simply don't possess the skills to navigate the course on our own. Too often it is when we are closest to our goal that we are most tempted to turn back in defeat. These are the moments when the Creator – the Universe, whatever power you wish to call it – invites us to ask for help, to receive the guides who can assist us in our journey.

A great deal of trust and surrender are involved when a person steps into unknown territory to explore the beautiful, hidden places that only a wise guide can show them. With the client's offering of trust comes the reciprocity of a guide's utmost care, a responsibility to protect the life of this stranger as well as her own. Together we are capable of reaching secret places that touch us to the depths of our soul; open our eyes to wonders previously unseen; and realize strengths we did not know we possessed. I picked the lines that delivered my client to his goal that day; but it was Eiji's undeterred faith in me that sealed our fate."[54]

JOURNAL ENTRY – CLIENT RELATIONSHIPS

Who are you in relation to your clients?
Do you accept invitations to Christmas parties or does that cross professional boundaries?
Have you sat with husbands or wives at squash tournaments or waited anxiously at the finish line for a client you helped train for an event?
Have you ever gone to a doctor appointment with a client?

Are you the ultimate source of all things fitness and wellness, or do your clients have wisdom to share with you as well?

What is your typical internal reaction or response to a client who is holding back out of fear?

Do you feel that the ability to empathize with your clients comes easily, or is there capacity to grow in this area?

Fears

The main objectives of my Sol Fitness Adventures are to *'challenge the body, lift the spirit, and engage the senses in wilderness.'* To many of my clients, dreams that used to seem unattainable suddenly become possibilities. I've learned that the courage a person cultivates by overcoming physical challenges in a controlled and safe environment can become the fire that fuels motivation and creates the resilience necessary to accomplish major life goals.

Part of challenging yourself is understanding what your fears are. Sometimes we don't even know a fear exists until we step out of our comfort zones and take on something new. I learned much about fear and chasing our dreams from a brave client who joined me on a four-day backpacking trip in the Zion backcountry and then on the Inca Trail in Peru. It isn't fun facing your fears, but, it is worth it!

I'm sure you've dealt with the fears your clients have related to their health and well-being. I remember training a client with a fear of heights who held her breath every time I pulled out the BOSU® ball. I watched as a grown man froze in fear and cried, terrified of stepping out onto a ledge to make his next move on a climb.

Maybe you've had a client with cancer, or who had knee surgery, or suffered a miscarriage. I think we mind/body specialists have well-developed stores of empathy compared to most people. Our bodies are experienced warriors, decorated with battle scars, perhaps a tattoo or two, and the inherent knowledge of overcoming obstacles and rising to meet physical challenge. Many of us may be fearless when it comes to learning a new sport or healing from injury.

JOURNAL ENTRY - FEARS

Warrior though you may be, what are you afraid of?
What happens if you get hurt on an outdoor fitness retreat and have to cancel clients?
How can you mitigate the risks?
What about aging, is it a far off impossibility or is there something your body is experiencing now that scares you?

Trips for the Bucket List

Sometimes it's uncomfortable to think about our own mortality, but it also gives us time to reflect on the beauty and wonder of this world. Think about the things you really want to accomplish and see in your finite time here on earth. Do you think you'll really go for it, or are you content to wait until everything is perfect to chase your dreams?

Most of the clients I guide on my fitness retreats are in the process of crossing an experience off their bucket list or intentionally experimenting to find out if the outdoor lifestyle is something they want to incorporate into their lives. It's a privilege and a lot of fun to be a part of their journey and provide some important guidelines and coaching. Watching my clients dig deep to make their dreams a reality and encouraging them through the setbacks has taught me a great deal about honoring where a person is on their journey.

It takes humility to accept when something doesn't go the way you all planned. One particular client, Sarah, comes to mind. (I've changed her name here). Her journey to test the boundaries of her comfort zone is one of my favorites and taught me a great deal about the complicated dynamics of working with people aspiring to accomplish big things in their fitness and outdoor life. This experience happened early on as I was experimenting with a variety of service offerings with Sol Fitness Adventures and saw my Adventure Travel Preparation service included in *Outside's* Top 10 list. While I've never published this short story anywhere else, I like to call this story *The Greatest Trip that Never Happened*.

The Greatest Trip That Never Happened

> Sarah was a 47-year old woman and mother of two young boys. She became friends with a group of super-fit and adventurous woman who convinced her to hike Mt. Kilimanjaro in Africa with them. A Pennsylvania native, Sara was not an outdoor

adventurer. Her idea of the outdoors was a nicely groomed beach in southern California or a walk in the city park!

With only six weeks to go before the trip, Sarah's husband, Mark, hired me to train her for the trek. She wasn't taking any time for herself and he was worried about her. I hadn't been to Kili – yet – but I'd read that it's a long slog of a hike to the top, that even one of the world's fittest have succumbed to high altitude sickness during their attempt to make the summit. Not content that mere gym workouts were up to the task, I designed a 6-week multifaceted training regimen to prepare Sarah for her quest. It wasn't enough to have high reserves of cardiovascular and muscular endurance. I wanted to help Sarah prepare mentally for the trip, to offer her the full gamut of sport-specific experiences that would give her a mental and emotional edge in hiking to 19,340 feet above sea level.

I called Sarah's program Mt. Kilimanjaro Adventure Training. She tackled strength training workouts 2-3 times a week. We hiked several times a week in the Santa Ynez Mountains in Santa Barbara, bought all of her gear (total cost was about $2,500), and scheduled her vaccinations – yellow fever, typhoid, hepatitis A, and diphtheria. The climax and my favorite part of her training program was a three-day high-altitude hiking trip to the Eastern Sierra, where she could experience what it felt like to hike all day and then have to sleep on the ground at night.

From our home base near June Lake we did three hikes with two major ascents. The first was a long but moderate hike in the Ansel Adams Wilderness to Devil's Postpile. The second day we hiked to the top of Mammoth Mountain at 11,053 feet. Both nights we put Sarah's new camping gear to the test and she slept like a baby – or so I thought – in a serene meadow next to the Owens River.

Our last day was an epic – we joined Sarah's adventurous friends on another full day hike to White Mountain Peak, elevation 14,252 feet above sea level. A mere 249 feet lower than Mt. Whitney, the tallest mountain in the lower 48 United States at 14,501 ft. The elevation of the trailhead alone was situated at 11,000 feet! The trail was long and rocky and it was Sarah's first time being that high in the atmosphere. Not knowing what it looked like that high up, she found the barren tundra landscape above treeline to be boring and ugly. In spite of the negatives Sarah's fitness levels were up to the challenge and we reached the summit in good time without any difficulty. Both physically and mentally, Sarah was ready for her trip.

But there was a problem.

Sarah's boys, 10 and 12 years old, had traveled often and loved to go to sleep-away camp. Sarah had never been the one to leave her boys at home while she traveled. Her youngest son researched the trip online and learned about the dangers of altitude sickness and began to have nightmares that his mother was going to die. Sarah began to lose sleep over it. During the last two weeks leading up to her trip to Kili, Sarah hadn't had more than four hours of sleep on any given night. She was tired, troubled and anxious.

A few nights before she was to leave for the trip Sarah invited me to a family meeting with her husband, Mark. I worried that the sleeplessness and anxiety, combined with the strain of high altitude, could combine into a dangerous cocktail, one that would, at the very least, ruin her trip, and at the worst result in serious injury. We agreed that if Sarah didn't go see a doctor for sleeping medication and get some rest before the trip, she should not go.

There's a deeper side to Sarah's story that I think is important to share. During our training I learned that Sarah was a spiritual woman. I took the risk of being too personal and asked if she'd prayed or meditated about her decision to hike Kili. She told me that she had been praying and trying to get a clear answer, but that she just felt confused and anxious. I shared that from my perspective that sounded like her answer – and the answer was 'No.'

Going to Africa without her husband and sons felt like a huge violation of who Sara was as a mother, a wife, and a woman. It didn't matter that she was in the comfortable position of being financially able to do anything she wanted to do. Hiking Kili without her family simply didn't fit into her value system.

Sarah was physically ready for the hike. I was proud of her hard work during training and I knew she'd do great if she decided to go. Going to Africa would be in violation of what was most important to her. Her integrity would be compromised; something that even the summit of one of the world's tallest peaks could not repair. I told her I would honor and respect her decision not to go if that's what she decided to do.

Sarah decided against going on the trip, and a few weeks later I received a letter thanking me for introducing her and her family to a new lifestyle. I couldn't have been more proud of a client. To this day I consider her Mt. Kilimanjaro Adventure Training one of my biggest successes.

Use this time to think about the places you dream to go. Your clients have these dreams of their own. Maybe you both imagine exploring the Andes Mountains by hiking the Inca Trail to Machu Picchu or stand up paddling the coast of Bali before doing yoga and meditating under a pagoda overlooking the sea. Your dreams and your client's dreams can be the material you use to lead your first fitness retreat. Take a moment to remember the places you dream to explore.

I wonder what kind of stories you'll create as you set off down this path? What's on your bucket list?

The Role of Play

Go Play Outside

The idea of play is an important one in terms of both behavioral and physical health. In a world that increasingly values hard work and progress, play often gets overlooked (and even repressed). I'm one of those people who has an insatiable appetite for play. My heart sank when I moved to Washington, D.C. in 2002 and could no longer 'play' outside in the wild ways I was accustomed to. If you're still on the fence about this topic or don't think I'm serious about the necessity of playing outside as a way to enhance our clients health and well-being, I invite you to sit for a moment with this thought from Brian Sutton-Smith, "The opposite of play is not work. It is depression."

Journal Entry – Go Play Outside

You're an adult and this is serious business, you tell me - surely I don't expect you to *play* and have *fun*! Surely I must be referring to your city-league softball or alumni kickball games. Oh, I know, maybe your idea of playing outside means running the same 3.5 mile loop every day between clients. I used to do that, trust me. If I could count the number of times I ran along the Potomac River to the Lincoln Memorial and back I'd be a rich lady. I know it's a run but come on, it isn't always fun!

> Were you ever told to 'go play outside' as a child?
> Have you ever watched a child play?
> Use this space to daydream about play and how you can incorporate more of it into yours and your clients' lives.

In Defense of Play

Behavioral scientists have found that children benefit immensely from being outdoors. In order to form a real and lasting connection and a feeling of safety, a child needs to be able to do what's called free play. Free play is unstructured time outdoors to play in the dirt, throw mud, build rock dams, collect bugs, talk to the plants, run through the sprinklers, to feel free and untethered. Louv found that kids who play outside show advanced cognitive development and spatial orientation. Symptoms of ADHD are improved after outdoor exposure. The outdoors develops increased resistance to negative stresses and depression.[55]

I've explored the outdoors with many children during my careers as a wildlife biologist and outdoor guide. Watching them play and run around like a small tribe is a joy to watch and a blast to interact with. Kids have an inherent curiosity of the natural world that can be infectious.

In 2013 I guided five trips of mixed families through southern Utah's National Parks. The families had never met and I wondered how the kids would get along. To my astonishment kids from across the country joined forces quickly and carelessly. They cheered each other on Class II rapids on the Colorado River in Moab. They put their arms around the one's who cried at the sight of a daddy-long-leg spider's nest in Secret Slot Canyon. Problems were solved quickly and diplomatically without me ever having to interject.

Play Defined

I've noticed that when parents are told things are good for their children, they'll prioritize the activities for the family around those things. When it comes to putting their own physical activities, hobbies, and health first, however, some parents feel a lot of guilt. I've spent this section presenting why the outdoors is great for kids because you'll be selling your clients on the idea, and it helps to have the facts.

The key is to help your adult clients make the connection that what's good for the kids'—playing outside—is just as good for them. Nature-based exercise not only builds physical fitness, it also strengthens our senses, our intellectual capacity, and our mental health. Louv's book *The Nature Principle* holds that a reconnection to the natural world is fundamental to human well-being. *Fundamental.* He goes on to explain that,

> "Play is something done for its own sake. It's voluntary, it's pleasurable, it offers a sense of engagement, it takes you out of time. And the act itself is more important than the outcome."[55]

What can you do today to reconnect with the natural world?
What physical activities or hobbies do you enjoy participating in outdoors?
When was the last time you asked a friend to go 'play?'
How do you play?

A Note on Journaling

Journaling allows you to understand you better!

Are you wondering why I asked all of these personal questions? Reflection is an important part of self-discovery, and self-discovery is one of the natural outcomes of Sol Guide Method and outdoor fitness retreats. Just as you spent time looking inward at yourself and your life, clients that join you on a retreat are on a quest to add more excitement, personal growth and satisfaction to their own lives. You'll watch as they naturally become more relaxed, happier, and more productive in their own lives. The journey of helping people discover not only new places, people, and activities, but also new dimensions of themselves is the payoff for venturing out of the indoor gyms and into *Mother Nature's Gym!*

The value of journaling as you read is not really in writing intricately detailed thoughts or amazing and perfectly worded responses. The journal entries are simply meant to be a personal recollection of your thoughts and ideas. Use them for what makes sense to you—as a form of personal development or to brainstorm, catalog and chart your progress toward leading your own outdoor fitness retreat.

JOURNAL ENTRY - PERSONAL JOURNALING

Do you currently keep a personal journal?
What value can journaling add to developing as a fitness professional and expanding your career opportunities?
Do you think you will recommend journaling to your clients?

Review – The Outdoor Fitness Guide

Multiple Choice

Complete the sentence by selecting the correct term or phrase.

1. Your job as a guide is to _____ lead your clients through an experience that has the potential to transform their lives.

    a. Quickly
    b. Quietly
    c. Blindly
    d. Safely

2. Which of the following is *not* one of your basic responsibilities when guiding an outdoor fitness retreat?

    a. Details like locations, start and end times, and emergency contact numbers
    b. Having alternative plans in case unexpected situations arise
    c. Making sure that all clients have taken their medications and have a working cell phone
    d. Awareness of local road and weather conditions

3. Exercises in intention-setting, mindfulness, and meditation help clients connect with their _____.

    a. Body
    b. Family
    c. Natural surroundings
    d. Flexibility

4. Which of the following statements is *not* true regarding children and play?

    a. Kids who play outside show advanced cognitive development and spatial orientation
    b. Children who spend a lot of time in natural settings outdoors tend to have more anxiety.
    c. Symptoms of ADHD are improved after outdoor exposure.
    d. The outdoors develops increased resistance to negative stresses and depression.

5. Free play is simply unstructured time outdoors to play in the dirt, throw mud, build rock dams, collect bugs, etc.

    a. True
    b. False

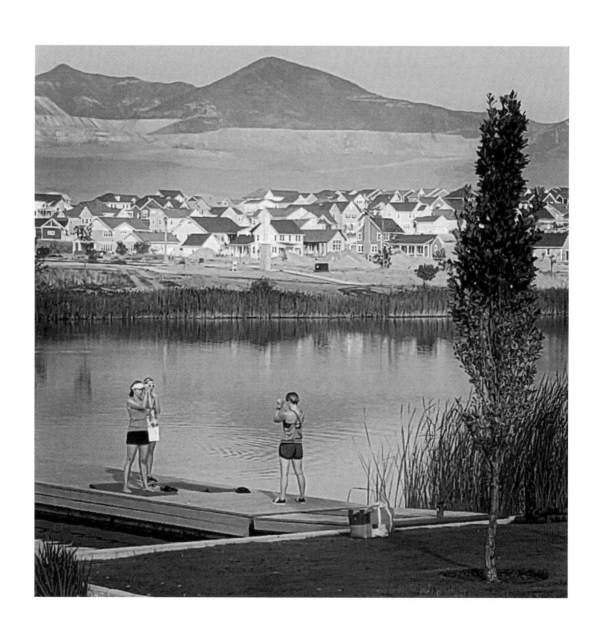

PART FIVE
CREATING OUTDOOR FITNESS RETREATS

"What happens after a missed opportunity, mistake, or failure is crucial. Those I coached didn't need to visualize success. Success would take care of itself if they took care of everything else. This included preparing for failure."

— JOHN WOODEN

Fitness Adventure Program Design

When an architect designs a building, he takes time to understand what the building will be used for, how people will interact in the space, the client's budget, and the client's expectations.

Similarly, when you design a fitness retreat for a client, you need to do so using the best information you have so that you and your clients are happy and everyone's expectations are met. In this lesson, you will learn how to gather the most important information and use it to plan your adventure. Specifically, you will learn:

- How to assess client needs and abilities
- How to choose the proper activities for a client
- How to program warm-ups and cool-down activities
- How to schedule your time

You have certain strengths and passions unique to your background, and your own programs will likely reflect those strengths and passions. That is good! No two adventure guides will provide the same experience. Choose to embrace your unique perspective on adventure fitness. It will help you find your niche in this market.

In today's world it's easy to book appointments via text or email without ever hearing each other's voices. The guide-client relationship is unique, so invest the time before the adventure to really understand the clients and their needs/desires. This is also the time to build the foundation for your relationship. You will have many types of clients; some will want to spend time getting to know you and will even become friends; others will prefer minimal personal interactions. As you spend time with the client in planning and designing the program, you will learn how to interact with them in a way that is most comfortable for you both. The chances of running a successful trip will be much higher as you make the time to connect in a more personal way before the adventure.

Client Intake and Assessment

The phrase '*Intake and Assessment*' sounds way too clinical for an outdoor fitness guide, but the idea is similar to the process of going to the ER when you have a sprained ankle. Before the doctor starts giving injections and prescribing medications they must take a patient through an intake and assessment process. Similarly, you will need to have important information from your clients ahead of time for the purposes of contracts, communication, and payment. You will also need a health history so you can understand any limitations or conditions a client may have that help you keep them safe.

Plan to include a proper intake and assessment of the client before you go to work planning the outdoor fitness retreat. This doesn't have to be performed in a formal, clipboard style fashion. You can easily cover this information in an email, a phone call, or an hour-long in-person meeting if possible. This process is comprised of the following three components:

1. Assess client abilities
2. Identify client objectives
3. Set clear expectations

Step One – Assess Client Abilities

The first step in designing a program is to **determine the fitness level and skill set of your clients**. If they're new clients, you can assess their fitness level by asking a few specific questions:

- How many times a week do you exercise?
- What kind of exercise do you do and for how long?
- What type of activity are you looking for now?
- Have you ever been advised by a doctor not to do certain exercises?
- What injuries have you suffered in the past?

Knowing your client's fitness level and their physical history is a great starting point. You can use a health history questionnaire to gather health information. This form asks your client specific questions about his/her health, both current and past. Having a written form is helpful because you can review the information as you design your fitness adventure. I explore health history questionnaires and their application to an outdoor setting in greater detail in *Adventures in MOTHER NATURE'S GYM The Business Manual.*

If you're planning a trip that you hope to offer to a group of clients, you *tell* them what the purpose of the trip is. For example, maybe you've introduced moon salutations to your yoga class. How cool would it be to do your moon salutation series under a full moon, after a sunset, on top of a cliff that you hike to? Wouldn't that experience give those heart openers a little more meaning?

Step Two - Identify Client Objectives

The next step in the process of designing a customized program is to **understand what the client wants to get out of their experience**. This requires you to ask a series of very direct questions and then listen carefully for anything you can read between the lines. For example, I have many prospective clients call me to say they want to go hiking in Zion National Park, and they heard I was "the person" to call. As you become the expert at leading fitness retreats in your area you can expect the same kind of phone call. Being "the person to call" is great, but when you really get to the heart of the matter, the adventure is not actually about me, or about you—it's about the client's journey and what they really want to get out of their adventure.

Rarely, but it does happen, clients can't verbalize exactly what it is they want out of their retreat, they've just heard from a friend that they 'should' do this or that or they 'must' visit such and such a location. That kind of ambiguity can make it incredibly difficult to meet expectations and can set you up for failure. In that case, you need to hone your conversation skills and get to the heart of what the client really wants.

As you read the questions below, imagine the discussion unfolding with a client. Visualize the specific locations and fitness adventures you plan to guide and insert them into the available spaces.

Location Specific - the following questions will help you understand where your adventure should take place:

> "So you've always dreamed of [what's your main adventure? Hiking, paddling, etc.] in [insert amazing location near you], fantastic!"

"What are the main features of [insert awesome venue] that you want to see?"

"Do you want to get off-the-beaten-path [what are the places only the local experts know about?] and away from other people or is it a bucket list adventure that you want to check off?"

Activity Specific - the following questions will help you understand what *activities* you should include:

"How much and what kind of exercise are you doing now?"

"Is [insert main activity of the place, hiking, paddling, etc.] something you've done before, or is this your first time?"

"Do you want to be challenged physically or does your body need a little R&R during this short vacation?"

"My specialty is combining [insert your mind/body discipline] with [what kind of adventure can you do in this place?]. Have you done [insert your mind/body discipline again] before?"

"I've found that doing [what do you do?] next to the lake at [what's the best time of day to be in your local outdoor venue?] is [insert adjective here: what's so special about this place? Is it restful, invigorating, spectacular, or spiritual?]. I'm excited for you to experience how it differs from indoors!"

Now you know your client's capabilities and what they expect to get out of the program. Next, you need to make sure everyone understands his or her role in the actual retreat.

Step Three – Set Clear Expectations

The third step in designing the fitness retreat is setting clear expectations. Your clients will likely come to you with very different experiences and views of fitness programs. This means that they all have different ideas about what their role is, what your role is, and how the professional relationship will work.

I once had a client say to me, while doing leg curls in a gym, "What's up with the poop-brown carpet? Is that the best they could get with all this money I pay each month?" Clients take a lot of pride in whom they choose to work with and where they choose to do it. Be prepared to have to answer for some aspects of the retreat that you may not have anything to do with, while taking control over the things that you do.

For example, if you have a client who has previously had a personal fitness instructor in a high-end corporate gym setting, that client may have the "client-is always-right" mentality. In that arena, the client probably *did* run the show. The client may think that the 7 a.m. Wednesday time slot is "their" time. They bought 30 sessions with the trainer, after all. Shouldn't that entitle the client to own their preferred hour of the day?

As you can imagine, the "client-is always-right" mentality won't work in the outdoor space. 'Out there' you don't have the umbrella of a large company covering your back if something goes wrong. 'Out there' many uncontrollable elements and inherent dangers exist.

Before you get 'out there,' you need to clearly convey your expectations to the client and listen carefully to their wants and needs. If there are misunderstandings, *now* is the time to iron those out . . . not out on the trail or on the river.

Just like in your indoor workspace, you have every right to tell the client what you expect of them. For example:

- Everyone must obey traffic laws while biking as a group on a busy road.
- Participants must drink one gallon of water throughout the hike on a 100-degree day.
- Paddlers must obey boat captain commands during a white water river trip.
- Skiers and snowboarders must not venture out of bounds or cut ropes.

Setting clear expectations:

- Keeps people safe
- Sets others at ease
- Positions you to be a respected leader
- Helps you run a successful outdoor fitness retreat

Answer the following questions to review what you've learned in this chapter so far.

Matching

Match the correct phrase to the appropriate step. Not all terms will be used.

What are the proper steps to follow when interviewing a new client? Match the phrase to the correct order, below.

Step 1 -   set clear expectations
Step 2 -   identify client objectives
Step 3 -   client assessment

Fill in the Blank

Select the word that best completes the paragraph from the list below. Not all terms will be used.

Client _____ and _____ helps you collect important information from _____ before the retreat for the purposes of communication, contacts, and _____ locations and difficulty levels. You will also need a _____ history so you can understand any _____ you may need to consider.

illnesses	vetting
assessment	payment
health	clients
political differences	intake
interviews	limitations

Structuring the Outdoor Fitness Retreat - FITT

Once the client intake and assessment (that sounds so formal!) is complete, you should begin to formulate a clear vision of the clients' wants, needs, and capabilities.

Next you'll shift your attention to the activities and the setting for your outdoor fitness retreat. How will you meet your clients' needs while challenging them but not pushing them beyond their limits? To accomplish this, we'll use the FITT method of program design.

FITT

The term *FITT* might be new to some of you. Personal trainers and group exercise instructors are probably familiar with FITT, a commonly used acronym in the fitness industry. The acronym stands for

- **F**requency
- **I**ntensity
- **T**ime
- **T**ype

Seasoned personal trainers will know that I didn't invent the FITT concept. Rather, in my 2014 article in IDEA Fitness Journal *Mother Nature's Gym*[56] I presented a basic outline of how to build upon this solid training foundation to create an outdoor fitness retreat. I'll take a deeper look into applying FITT in the sections that follow.

Frequency

Creating the structure around your outdoor fitness retreat begins with the principle of frequency. Frequency refers to how often your clients will engage in the planned activities and is a rate of occurrence. You can consider frequency in daily, weekly, monthly, quarterly, or yearly terms. Ask yourself the following questions:

- How often are your clients interested in getting outdoors?
- What will their time allow them to commit to?
- How will the outdoor fitness retreat compliment your indoor practice?
- How often can you reasonably run a retreat and add to rather than take away from your existing training revenue stream?

There are no right answers to these questions. Your availability and your clients interest and commitment levels will dictate when and how often you plan an outdoor adventure.

I recommend starting out slow. Talk to your clients about their availability. Is there a day or time that works best? Plan a nearby outdoor event with at least one month's notice. Emphasize that they'll apply the techniques they're working on in the studio to a practical, real life setting. Encourage them to come out and meet your other clients and make new friends. Test your retreat on a small scale before expanding to bigger and better plans.

Understanding Frequency

A great way to start is to take a look at the "big picture" of your client's programming. When I'm training I usually have similar themes I'm working on with everybody, even if each individual session might be tailored to the individual or the class needs. Within that big picture there is an ideal point at which it would be both fun and affirming to test the waters with a real-life scenario outside.

ACTIVITY

Here's one example of how to integrate outdoor fitness retreats into your training practice, and how to show clients measurable results:

EXAMPLE

Say you're a personal trainer on a real Bosu® kick, or a Yoga instructor who emphasizes single legged balance positions Yoga. At the early phases of the balance programming you may want to plan a stand up paddle fitness retreat to get a gauge on what baseline balance is for your clients and how it differs across the age and fitness level spectrum. You could make the retreat fun and social, include prizes and giveaways from local sponsors and invite everyone to bring their significant others or children.

During the retreat you'll be able to watch everyone's abilities (or lack thereof). You'll return to the gym and studio and continue training, knowing that there is a second follow-up event planned in six weeks where everyone can go back and try paddling again. Armed with the knowledge of who needs what, you'll be able to fine-tune the workouts before the next retreat. It's very likely that you and your clients will see an improvement in their performance on the water the second time around.

The real life application of demonstrating measurable progress reinforces the value you provide in your training. You've just exposed clients to a fun outdoor activity that they've probably wanted to try, but just hadn't got around to yet. The bonus should be that you've been able to make a bit of extra money doing something you enjoy.

Now, revisiting the frequency of the SUP retreats, if you were to space them one week apart, would you expect to see the improvement in their second paddle session? You may see a little bit of improvement, sure. Will it be a direct result of the training you've done with them in the gym during the last week? No, because you haven't given their body enough time to create the neural pathways, muscular strength, and flexibility that optimize physical performance.

If you think strategically about how frequently you want to produce an outdoor fitness retreat, you can really leverage them to your advantage. I suspect that once you do the first one you'll have a good idea of how frequently you're willing to incorporate fitness retreats into your business model.

Take a moment to reflect on the themes or elements of your training practice, either what it is right now or what the emphasis will be as the periodization process continues.

How long will each training phase last?
How often can you run an outdoor fitness retreat for maximum effect?
How often do you have the extra time and energy required to organize and lead a retreat?

Intensity

Remember, the ultimate goal of leading an outdoor fitness retreat is for people to have a good time out there! For some people that might mean engaging in an all out suffer-fest. Others will prefer to be pushed up to and not one step beyond their comfort zone. I dare say that many people don't even know what their body is capable of! Your job is to design an experience that fits everyone attending the retreat perfectly.

The work you have done with intake and assessment will help you understand the correct intensity level for each of your clients. There are other considerations as well. Similar to exercise and machine selection when training indoors, when you guide an outdoor fitness adventure you not only have to consider the fitness level of your client, but match it to the perfect type of terrain as well.

Below are some examples of questions you might ask yourself:

1. Do you plan to hike a steep or rocky mountain grade?
2. What class rapids do you plan to kayak?
3. How wide is the shoulder of the road on the route you plan to road bike?
4. Is the trail maintained or will it require an element of bushwhacking?

One of the difficulties in leading outdoor adventures is selecting a venue that will be appropriate for everyone. This is easy to do with small private groups and individuals because they probably already know and support one another, or they know how to push and encourage each other in just the right way.

Matching fitness levels with the right venue becomes more of a challenge as the size of the group grows. For example, I know that for every six people I take stand up paddleboarding there will be two people who struggle and fall in, regardless of water conditions.

Another great example is skiing. You may have a top age-ranked triathlete who is a true specimen of physical condition but has never been on skis before. If you were to pair that athlete up with an overweight person with bad knees who has skied his whole life, who do you think is going to perform better? The overweight person with bad knees will perform better on skis than the triathlete, every time. Why? Because fitness, skill levels, and fear thresholds are different for everyone, and the training principle of specificity means the body adapts to it's specific training environment.

As you craft the intensity of your outdoor fitness retreat, keep the following three factors relating to intensity in mind:

1. Consider both fitness and skill level
2. Select outdoor venues that provide a safe challenge
3. Highlight client capabilities

Step One – Consider both fitness and skill level

The higher the precision of movement required, the more likely it is that you'll group people based on skill level rather than fitness level. From that baseline, divide clients into groups of beginner, intermediate, and expert skill levels. If everyone is a beginner, you might consider forming groups according to fitness or overall conditioning levels.

EXAMPLE

Cycling is a great sport for all fitness levels. It's quite easy to find terrain that is both fun to ride and beautiful to look at. It's quite obvious that the steeper and longer the hill, the more cardiovascular fitness and muscular strength your client needs to get to the top.

There's another factor that is equally as important as the terrain—the clients' familiarity with a road bike. Have they ever used clip in pedals before? If not, remember that there's a learning curve and you can expect a few falls. Best not to learn on an adventure with a bunch of experts, that's a great way to intimidate your client!

Then you have to think about the gears. Road bikes don't have as many gears as a mountain bike. The gear system is different on every bike, and if you're renting, the client has to learn quickly how to get into the right gear. I'm always surprised when I catch up to a client struggling to get up a hill who has simply forgotten to switch to their easier gear! How could they forget? They do forget, or freeze in fear, and get scared that they'll make a mistake and drop their chain, or worse—break the bike!

You have to send the time before anyone even sits on a bike to review the bike components, teach proper bike handling/riding technique, and review the rules of the road. Plan to review them often. Plan to have to ride up to a client and insist that they get out of the road. Be firm when you have to, but remind people that it's all right to make mistakes. Make this outdoor fitness retreat as safe and fun a learning environment as possible for your clients (I've found that planning a 'car stop' with treats and cold drinks is a great way to keep things fun!).

Step Two – Select outdoor venues that provide a safe challenge

It's very easy to get in over your head "out there." That said, it's just as easy not to. You must take the time to do your due diligence. Always do a "pre-trip" visit to the venue to test, inspect, and experience the location and activity yourself before you show up with a group of clients. Only then will you be prepared to anticipate what could go wrong and to convey the intensity of the activity to clients.

EXAMPLE

Lake Powell, in the Glen Canyon National Recreation Area on the Utah/Arizona border is one of my favorite places to lead fitness and stand up paddle retreats. With over 2,000 miles of shoreline, the lake is an enormous wonderland of exploration. If you've never been there, all the rock cliffs start to look the same after a while and it can be difficult to orient yourself.

On day trips I like to transfer everyone by boat to a particular cove called Ice Cream Canyon, teach the dry-land stand up paddle or kayak lesson, and then lead everyone out onto the water for practice. Now I know to direct paddlers to the left where the cove turns into a dead end box canyon and forces them to turn around and return to where we started. If they go to the right, the cove opens up to the main lake where there is plenty of boat traffic and many more fingers and canyon offshoots.

From out on the main lake it's very easy to get lost. Want to guess how I figured this out? You got it—one day I assumed people knew better than to paddle out into the open lake, and that if they did it was easy enough to get back. When the husbands of the two women who went joy-paddling into open water told me their wives had been missing for an hour, guess who got to go looking? Sure enough, they'd been chatting and forgotten where they were. A boater picked them up and drove them into the marina, where they sat and had ice cream while the rest of us were frantically searching for them.

Step Three – Highlight client abilities

There's a fine line between providing just the right level of challenge and watching someone have an epic fail. Don't flirt with that line and please don't make the adventure about you. Set your clients up for success in every way by designing outdoor fitness retreats that highlight clients' physical capabilities rather than diminish them. Then sit back as they tell all their friends how great you are, send you their referrals, and come back for more.

EXAMPLE

I once had a super fit couple from New York City hire me to plan their outdoor fitness retreat to Southern Utah's National Parks. Each day we'd do a core warm up, hike about six to ten miles, and then stretch and meditate afterward.

As we talked on our first day in Zion National Park, they mentioned that they'd always dreamed of rock climbing and rappelling but had never had the chance to try it outside. I watched how agile and fearless they moved on one of our most challenging hikes—straight up, with chains because of steep drop offs. Both physicians, they were able to think through obstacles they encountered and adjust easily, without emotional reactions.

As luck would have it, Zion National Park is one of the best places in the world for canyoneering—where you use a rope to lower yourself over a cliff to explore deeper and deeper into a canyon. It so happens that, Zion being my area of expertise, I happen to know the best climber and canyoneer guide in the state of Utah, and I've explored many of the slot canyons in the area with him. I knew from watching the New Yorkers hike that they had the mental and the physical ability to navigate the next level of challenging terrain.

I called my friend Dan that night and the next day and we hired him to guide us safely through a spectacular canyon with 11 rappels, three of them into deep water. The level of difficulty was perfect for them and they had an amazing time. I dare say it was the highlight of their entire trip.

Time

The first 't' in the acronym FITT stands for time, which applies to program design in three different ways:

1. Length of each individual aspect of the outdoor fitness retreat
2. Periodization, or introducing the activity at the proper point in the training program
3. Duration of the retreat as a whole

We'll look at each one of these aspects of time individually, below.

Length of Time for Each Individual Outing

How do you know how long an outdoor fitness retreat should last? You will find it relatively easy to determine the length of time for each aspect once you are familiar with your client's capabilities and prior experiences.

What about for new clients? The first bout for beginners, whether it be the fitness workout or the outdoor sport or activity, should be no longer than 90 minutes. This concept is explained by basic principles of motor learning. A person learning a new movement pattern will make maximum progress only up to a certain point. Once that threshold is crossed you'll yield diminishing returns.

Motor learning studies have shown that the body learns new movement patterns best when spread out across a number of days or shorter bouts rather than one long, concentrated learning period. The brain works in a very systematic way when it comes to learning, whether its cognitive information or sport-specific movement patterns. The cerebellum, the prefrontal cortex and the hippocampus all play roles in processing and storing executive functions and motor movements. Fundamental patterns of thinking and movements that are automatic and second nature are stored in the basal ganglia, cerebellum, and brain stem—subconscious areas that free up space and allow the brain to continue adapting.[57]

Of course, experts can progress to longer sessions and even sport-specific multi-day trips. Keep it short and sweet for the beginners to guarantee that they have a great experience.

I once had a new client asked me to teach her how to stand up paddle. She had a lake trip coming up in one month and she wanted to learn how to paddle so that she could maximize her time on vacation. While she was deconditioned and slightly overweight, she was a former ballet dancer and had a high level of kinesthetic awareness.

After a few workouts and plenty of requests from her, I consented to take her paddling. It was a disaster. I hadn't worked with her long enough to know the extent to which her tight calves restricted movement at her ankles. She was unable to flatten her feet on the board in order to stand up from the beginner kneeling position, and the shoreline didn't allow us to start from a standing position.

How often do you have a client in the gym try to stand on only one leg at a time from a quadruped (all fours) position? Well, it would have been a wise move to try indoors before I took her out on the water. She made many attempts to stand but kept falling off the board, and her weight made it very difficult to get back on the board. She felt frustrated, self-conscious, and quickly became physically exhausted. It was a disaster and I felt terrible about it.

Introducing the Activity at the Proper Point in Training

As you work with a client, you become familiar with their strengths and weaknesses and you communicate better with one another. As you learn about your client, you will be better able to judge when is the right time in your program to introduce an activity. Sometimes it is common sense, for example, you don't take someone stand up paddling without a life jacket unless you know they can swim (don't do it anyway, by the way!). Other times, you really have to consider how the client will be able to apply his/her skills to a new activity.

I could have prevented the paddleboarding ballerina disaster I described earlier if I had remembered to introduce the outdoor activity at the appropriate time, how? By performing the proper assessment of her strength and mobility in the indoor studio setting where we trained twice weekly. Instead of telling her that she wasn't ready and working on the flexibility and strength that would set her up for success, I gave in to the pressure and set her up to fail. It was a valuable lesson and a mistake I learned from.

Duration of the Fitness Retreat

Variety is important to most clients. Obviously, no one likes to be bored, and with the constant distraction of technology at our fingertips, it's been said that our attention spans are getting shorter. When you create outdoor fitness retreats with multiple components, you need to consider time in yet a different way.

> **IMPORTANT!**
>
> If your adventure features multiple physical activities, such as the concepts introduced in Sol Guide Method, you'll need to consider the length of each individual activity as it relates to the overall duration of the day. For example, you may plan a day that starts with a core workout, leads into a hike and meditation at a spectacular mountain overlook, and ends with a hike back out followed by a stretch, and then perhaps a nice meal. While each activity alone may be short in duration, the retreat as a whole could turn into a horrendously long day for others. Make sure you not only structure, but also communicate timeframes clearly with your client – and then stick to it.

It's helpful to give the client an overview at the beginning so they know what to expect. Be prepared to be flexible. Have an alternate route or activity in mind in case someone gets tired. Someone might pay you for a three-hour guided outdoor fitness adventure; but you must stop if after two hours their performance starts to decline, before they get hurt.

Type

The type of outdoor activity is typically at the top of the list when planning an outdoor fitness retreat - probably because it's the most fun. This is where you can get creative and combine your passion for fitness and the outdoor sports you love. Once you know how to match the frequency, intensity, and time principles of program design to individual fitness levels, it will be easy to choose the type of activity.

What Type of Outdoor Fitness Retreat Is Best for Your Client?

You may have particular clients in mind when designing your outdoor fitness retreat, and that will make it easy to choose which outdoor activity you include. If you're just interested in creating an experience that will attract your clients and help them enjoy cultivating their health and wellness with nature, the type of retreat you plan is the million-dollar question.

One good starting point that's easy to overlook is to simply ask questions - lots of questions. Ask your clients what they like to do. Do they watch with envy as you leave for a ski trip each winter? What are (or were) they really great at before they got pinned down to a profession? The more questions you ask, the more information you will have to create something truly unique and fun.

Three other important factors that influence the type of fitness retreat you create include seasonality, local recreation spots, and indoor training goals.

Seasonality

Depending on where you live, the adventure you choose may change with the seasons. Perhaps you want to plan a ski fitness trip during the winter quarter. Maybe you live in a location ideal for water sports, making summer the ideal time of year. The point is, you want the outdoor component of your outdoor fitness retreat to align with the time of year that offers the most enjoyment for your clients.

Winter sports include snowshoeing, skiing, snowboarding and cross-country skiing. Water sports like open water swimming, surfing, kayaking, and stand up paddling are always refreshing during hot summers months. Spring and fall, what we call shoulder seasons in Utah, are perfect for hiking, cycling, and exploring deep canyons.

If you live within a few hours of a ski resort, and I realize not everyone does, winter is a great time to plan a fun fitness adventure for your clients. Let everyone make their own travel arrangements. You can call the resort ticket office and inquire about group sales. Plan a 15-minute warm up at the base. Hire a group ski instructor from the resort for first-timers and spend the day on the slopes. Agree on the time and place to meet for lunch and spend the afternoon skiing together. End the day with a good stretch, hot chocolate, soak in the hot tub and some s'mores and hot toddies. Fun!

Local Recreation Spots

What unique geological features are near your community? What are the awesome outdoor venues in your state or region that every one of your clients needs to visit? I live in northern Utah, and I'm still shocked when I meet clients who've never visited the National Parks in our own backyard. Sometimes people just need a reason, or a group to join. Go ahead and give them one!

Take some time to research places that are within striking distance. Often state parks and historical locations are hidden treasures that offer great scenery.

I don't care where you live in the world - whether it's the most densely populated urban environment on the planet or in the middle of rural farmland – there's bound to be an urban park somewhere within city limits or a wide and beautiful landscape to explore on the outskirts of town. You owe it to yourself and your clients to get out there and enjoy it! When I lived in Washington, D.C. I would often drive 30 minutes to escape the city and hike the Billy Goat Trail on the Potomac River with my clients. It was a godsend.

Indoor Training Goals

You probably have clients that fall into certain age groups or activity levels. Many of my older clients or those with knee and ankle injuries like to work to improve their balance. The middle-aged business types are usually into trying new things and have the money to get after it like a true weekend warrior. Younger clients are still pushing their limits and developing healthy habits. They also tend to have less money to play with. These are all generalizations, of course, but what I'd like you to consider is whether you want to design outdoor fitness retreats that appeal to everyone across the age spectrum - or target one main demographic.

What type of retreat would complement your clients' indoor training programs? Think about the movement patterns and objectives you focus on in the studio and design an experience that will amplify and highlight their progress. Or think of the retreat as cross training and include an outdoor activity that is completely different and new. It's up to you!

EXAMPLE

One of the most targeted, specific examples of aligning an outdoor fitness retreat with an indoor training routine is swimming. If you have swimmers or triathletes among your clients they most likely spend an awful lot of time in an indoor pool. What if you could arrange for a swim instructor or triathlon coach to meet your group at a lake or the ocean for a few hours of open water swim technique? You can warm up with dry land training before the swim and finish up with breathing and stress reduction exercises on the shoreline after. Hire a food truck or cater a picnic for the icing on the cake. What a great outdoor fitness retreat!

Matching

Match the correct term or word to the corresponding letter in the FITT acronym.

1. Intensity   a. F
2. Type   b. I
3. Frequency   c. T
4. Time   d. T

Multiple Choice

Circle the letter that corresponds to the correct answer for each question, below.

1. What is the ideal length of time of an outdoor activity for a beginner?

    a. 60-minutes
    b. 90-minutes
    c. Three hours
    d. Four hours

2. What are the three factors that influence the type of outdoor fitness adventure you design?

    a. Seasons
    b. Local politics
    c. Local hot spots
    d. Training goals

3. Which of the following would *not* be considered an ideal activity for someone interested in a water sports fitness retreat?

    a. Sea kayaking
    b. Open water swimming
    c. Hiking a rain forest during the rainy season
    d. Stand up paddling
    e. Snorkeling

4. Select the three factors that influence the intensity level of an outdoor fitness retreat:

    a. Fitness and skill level
    b. Group dynamics
    c. Time of year
    d. Activities designed to highlight clients' physical capabilities
    e. Proximity to water

Intuitive Training

Now that you've reviewed the program design principles of FITT, it's a good time to talk about training from an intuitive vantage point. Intuitive refers to making a decision based on how something feels, rather than based on conscious reasoning. Most of us naturally fall into the category of being either more intuitive or more "heady." It takes work to balance the two and make good decisions.

I was initially a very regimented personal trainer because I came into my fitness career from the textbook-heavy background of a science major at a university. I became even more analytical as I earned additional certifications and learned the methods that my employers wanted me to implement with my clients. Add to that corporate liability, where trainers are required to keep detailed records of client training, and I was stuck in the cycle of pre-planning and executing exacting workouts. It got to the point where it just wasn't fun anymore. I quit growing professionally and my training became stagnant.

Changing venues was exactly what I needed to grow as a trainer. Some clients came with me; others didn't. I was forced to change my methods, which was incredibly stimulating. I threw away the clipboard and found myself in training sessions where the client trusted me to lead the way based on what I saw and *felt*. Of course I still applied the basic programming methods of FITT, along with all the other learned training fundamentals. Rather than dictate the session based on my clipboard of pre-planned exercises, I began to *feel* what to ask the client to do next. Sometimes what happened in the moment was radically different than what I planned going into the session.

One of my colleagues in Washington, D.C. taught me a few simple thought processes that helped me continue to evolve into the intuitive teacher I am now. One of the questions is, "what would feel good next?" In other words, rather than think strictly in terms of opposing muscle groups or dictated exercise sequences, how can I ask the body to move in a way that feels good to my client?

Another similar question to ask yourself is "how can I continue to apply pressure in this same direction in a way that ultimately reaches muscle fatigue, failure, or frustration?" The goal, of course, is to help the client reach greater strength and fitness levels. As a teacher you accomplish this by approaching a session with a planned course of action in mind, while at the same time being prepared to change course based on what you actually see happen in the client's body.

Let me give you a concrete example. To accomplish the goal of improving strength within a 55-minute training session you need to methodically increase the difficulty of the workout. I'll share an example in an exercise sequence—and the thought process behind it—that does just that:

- Prone (face down) Pilates swimmer
- Plank
- Push up
- Bent over row
- Triceps extension from bent over row

Can you see a pattern as you break down the exercise sequence? Now, let me give you a few additional questions to consider regarding this exercise sequence. That's five exercises in a row with the client facing the floor. Do you think increasing muscle tension will build up in the posterior chain this sequence of exercises? Is the client going to start getting a little edgy during this sequence? Am I affecting change in the muscle groups with this cycle?

Now, what am I, the personal trainer thinking? How do I use my intuition to respond to what's happening in the very moment my client is performing these exercises? By being right there with them, I make on the spot adjustments to the number of reps or the length of time I require them to do each exercise. I instruct the client to keep going until I literally see fatigue coming on, and then tell them to do 5-10 more reps. If I don't see signs that I'm taxing their body by that 4th or 5th exercise, guess what? I'm going to keep piling it on, either by immediately repeating the set with heavier weight, more reps, and longer durations of each set, or with a whole new set of floor-facing exercises.

Designing the Workouts

As you design the workouts for your fitness retreat, think about how the exercises you select will complement the overall movement pattern of the day. Use the FITT principles to guide your thought process but remember to allow yourself to be intuitive and make changes when you're in the moment.

The Body-Weight Exercise Arsenal presented in Part Six is a compilation of functional movements that are grouped into clusters. As you design your retreat you can use the exercises like you would a toolbox with interchangeable parts—one exercise can go in any cluster, and any cluster can go with any activity.

The included basic warm-up and relaxation exercise clusters can be used with any activity and perform the dual functions of warm ups and cool downs.

KEY TERMS

Posterior Chain - Refers to the muscles and connective tissue that comprise the posterior, or back side of the body. Includes everything from the ankles up to the neck.

Functional exercises - those designed to improve the performance of everyday, real-life movements.

Equipment and Props

If you're a personal trainer coming from a traditional studio or gym setting, you may find that training on a Yoga mat in the outdoors, without the accoutrement of equipment and toys, is a real challenge. Similarly, Yoga and Pilates instructors may be wary of breaking from your protocols and instructing in a more functional, strength type of method.

Keep in mind that your client may feel vulnerable as well, stripped of the weights, machines, and classrooms full of people to hide beyond. And the mirrors? Now nobody can see what they're doing! This is an opportunity for you (both) to be creative. Go back to the basics of everyday movement to deliver an effective workout using nothing but the bare minimum.

The exercises used in my Sol Guide Method of outdoor fitness retreats (1/2-day and one-day adventures) are performed using only bodyweight. Of course, there are endless possibilities to progress the exercises using a few simple props that you can throw in your car or backpack. These props include bands and tubing, TRX Suspension Training® and Rip Trainers™, Pilates circles, Gliding discs, stability and weighted balls, speed ladders, hand weights, jump rope, cones, Bosu® balls and countless more.

In the Body-Weight Exercise Arsenal chapter you will learn how to choose bodyweight exercises and how to perform them. You will also learn which exercises work well with which outdoor activities. You can add these to your own personal exercise arsenal.

Obviously, I've shared my methods and favorite exercises here. What's most important is that you stay within your comfort level and area of expertise. What I want to challenge you to do is think outside the box and select the exercises that compliment the outdoor activity (i.e. cycling, hiking, swimming, stand up paddling, etc.). You're preparing to leave the traditional indoor gym, yoga, and Pilates studios – what kind of exercises do you want to choose?

Equipment that travels well:

- Bands and tubes
- TRX Suspension Training®
- Rip Trainers™
- Pilates circles
- Gliding discs
- Stability balls and weighted balls
- Speed ladders
- Hand weights
- Jump rope
- Cones
- Bosu® balls

New Clients on a Fitness Retreat

At some point during my time training clients in gyms and studios, I realized that I felt hindered by the institutional feel and restrictions the setting imposed. That's when I began to fuse my knowledge and passions. I applied what I learned as a wildlife biologist and environmental consultant to what I knew about physical and mental wellness. The end result was my boutique tour operator business Sol Fitness Adventures.

Training in the studio and learning new thought processes was great preparation for what I do now with my customized outdoor fitness retreats. I now work primarily with travelers to Utah. Most of these travelers have their own trainers and yoga instructors back home. For whatever reason - the destination, the outdoor component, the promise of a vacation tailored to their specific health and wellness goals, or even my reputation - something prompted them to hire me to plan and lead their outdoor fitness retreat.

Sometimes, if my guests are staying at a spa, I do use the weight room with my guests. It depends on their goals. More frequently I'm leading workouts in *Mother Nature's Gym*—the natural surroundings where my guests have said they want to explore. Most resorts and hotels have great outdoor patios and spaces that make fantastic core workout and meditation settings. I like to find somewhere private for a full core workout, but clients are usually comfortable warming up and cooling down in large open spaces.

You may choose to work only with your existing clients as you get started leading your own outdoor fitness retreats. In that case, you'll already know exactly how to train their bodies. If you offer your fitness retreats to a wider audience, you'll need to get comfortable working with bodies you've never encountered before. This requires a keen eye and understanding of movement patterns, an arsenal of exercises at your disposal, and the willingness to be flexible and spontaneous. With experience you'll come to trust yourself more, settling into an intuitive rhythm of training that feels good and yields great responses from your client.

When you have new clients on a fitness adventure, you will want to:

- Have a keen eye. Pay attention to what you see and feel and hear the client say.
- Understand healthy basic movement patterns—and recognize those that aren't.
- Have a large collection of exercises in your mental toolbox that you can select from.
- Be flexible and spontaneous, willing to alter your course.
- Have a backup plan in case of bad weather or unforeseen circumstances.

Fill in the Blank

Using the words listed on the left enter the correct word in the appropriate space. Not all terms will be used.

1. Working with new clients requires understanding _____, an _____, and _____.
2. Mother Nature's Gym consists of the _____ of the _____ of a _____.
3. Mastering the art of the workout requires equal amounts of _____ and a highly developed _____.
4. Add _____ and increase _____ to a workout by adding props and _____.

movement patterns	cardio
spontaneity	intuition
nutrition patterns	education
arsenal of exercises	workout designs
location	portable equipment
fitness retreat	resistance
natural surroundings	distance
physical building	difficulty

Case Study: A Cycling Adventure

I've covered a lot of information in this lesson about outdoor fitness retreat program design. Now let's take a look at how the concepts you've learned are applied to half and full day fitness adventures.

Often a retreat is multi-sport, but typically there is one main event. Here I want to share with you what it looks like to plan, host, and run a cycling fitness adventure. Sure, anyone can go ride a bike, but not everybody does. Believe it or not, not everyone learned how to ride a bike when they were kids. Further, the idea of putting on all that spandex and clipping into pedals can be terrifying to a lot of people! You can make this a fun coaching experience by taking the time to work with the clients in a safe and controlled situation on a spin bike first, then segue into an actual bike ride outside.

REMEMBER

The term *customized* means that no adventure will be just like another. Every experience will be custom-fit to match the fitness and skill levels of your guests. Hey, isn't that funny? Sounds very similar to creating a personal fitness training or private yoga or Pilates session, doesn't it? That's right, you already know how to do this!

I'll share with you a specific cycling fitness retreat that I led for eight women on the Central Coast of California. A friend from the adventure travel industry referred the trip leader – the organizer of the friend group - to me. We talked about her goals and vision for the trip and emailed back and forth until we had the right location for the time of year and level of difficulty dialed in.

The group ranged in age from 63–70 years old, all fit and active. Some had traveled the world on cycling trips while one woman had never ridden a bike – so she trained for our retreat exclusively in spin classes. Several of the women were afraid to wear clip pedals and used flat pedals instead (never use cages!). Two women brought their own bikes and I made arrangements for the other six women to rent. Each person was on an individual quest, but all had a great time supporting the others in the group. Me and my co-guide , a personal trainer and triathlete from Austin, Texas, thoroughly enjoyed our time with this group of friends.

Take a dive into the next few pages for the full breakdown and flow of a day on the trip. I've also included a Journal Entry, so you can begin thinking about your own cycling fitness retreat. Where have you always wanted to go?

A Day's Schedule

Now let's look at the schedule I designed for the first day of the California cycling fitness retreat (the actual trip was five days). Adding the fitness component is a unique approach to a single-day cycling adventure, something the average cycling trip tour operator doesn't know how to do.

7 a.m. — Breakfast: Certainly not required but this is a nice way to gather the group and to make sure that they eat before the ride. You can host this at your favorite local coffee shop or the closest picnic spot to the beginning of the ride with a simple trip to the grocery store. Include the cost in the overall price of the trip or offer it as an add-on or 'on your own' feature that adds value.

8:30 a.m. — Warm-up: This is the time to prepare the body for movement, to let the body help relax the mind, and to build a fun group dynamic between your clients (who may not have met each other before). Be sure to do this somewhere quiet and protected from traffic. On the grass or a corner of the parking lot can work just fine.

I like to start with some fun ice-breaker activities to make people smile. You can form a circle and have everyone scratch the name of their neighbor onto their back. Switch directions and do a quick shoulder rub or choppy-choppy or back scratch. If you really want to mess with people bring the circle in tight and ask them to give their neighbor an elbow hug, sound goofy? Try it and see!

Once you've broken the ice and helped people become comfortable, it's time to draw from your arsenal of body-weight exercises for the core workout. You can use the exact sequence presented in Part Six of this course or make up your own, but remember the objective is to warm up the large muscle groups, *not* stretch and relax them. This is not the time for yoga—save that for *after* the ride. Spend 30-minutes to one hour on this part of the day, depending on how much time you've budgeted for the event.

9:30 a.m. — Time for the safety talk: This is when you explain to the clients what to expect on their ride. It's always great to share a map of the area, whether digitally or printed, to help people orient themselves. You may even consider printing the map and route notes out so that each person has his or her own copy during the ride. You can print this on Rite In The Rain paper to make the notes weatherproof.

There are a number of safety measures to talk through before anybody gets on the bike. I discuss safety measures in great detail in *Adventures in MOTHER NATURE'S GYM The Business Manual*, the accompaniment to this book.

9:45 a.m. — Distribute route notes: The best way to keep everyone on track and combat the reality of the group spreading out is to prepare typed and detailed route notes. To do this often requires a fair amount of what we call 'pre-trip planning.' To create route notes, you will literally drive the route, carefully taking notes of each mile marker that signifies a change in direction or significant landmark. Most rental shops now equip bikes with GPS units to sync mileage. Of course you can use apps such as Strava and others, but don't let these replace your own preparation of route notes for the group.

12:30 p.m. — Post ride stretch: It usually takes about 15 minutes after the ride finishes to collect everyone from the restroom and for the banter to subside. This is the time to gather everyone together again for a little TLC.

Flexibility training can take many forms, and as you're probably aware, there are various professional opinions and viewpoints about stretching. Here's where I stand on this issue: flexibility training feels good. So whether you choose 15-second static stretches, partner stretches, or active relaxation, do something that helps everyone's heart rate return to normal and their body feel good.

Lunch: If you're in an area with outdoor seating it's fun to go straight to lunch after the ride. Some people may prefer a quick shower before lunch, but I've seen billionaires sit and enjoy a great sandwich, spandex and all. Including lunch is another way for you to add value to your adventure. Estimate the cost, add 10-15% for your profits and don't forget the tip, and you pick up the tab for everyone. They'll be glad they didn't have to worry about carrying wallets and money on the ride!

Afternoon: Clients love to be pampered. If you've planned a full day activity, reserve the afternoon for bodywork appointments. Depending on the size of the spa, many can work on up to four people at a time. While the first four are getting worked on, the other four are relaxing in the spa, playing cards or learning to change a flat bike tire. There are so many ways to add value to your clients experience and treat them to an adventure they'll always remember.

After the ride finishes is an excellent time for breathing and guided visualization exercises as well. You can take advantage of the quieted state of mind that the biking has induced and lead the clients into a very relaxed mindset.

Encourage your clients to drink a lot of water during the post ride activities and have snacks readily available as soon as they step off the bike. Prepare a cooler full of chilled hand towels for wiping the sweat off their brows, and if you really want to impress, infuse the towels with a lavender or eucalyptus essential oil. It's pure bliss!

JOURNAL ENTRY – CYCLING FITNESS RETREAT SAFETY TALK

What kind of road surfaces will they run into?
Are conditions wet or dry?
How close should they ride to the others in the group?
How will you communicate with each other?
Did you rent bikes or is everyone on their own?
If you rented, do a review of the gears and breaks. Make sure seat heights are the proper fit. Check that helmets are securely fastened. Do you have reflective lights or clothing in the group?

Planning for Success

The key to success for a half-day or full-day cycling adventure is in your organization. **Have a plan and know your timelines**. Keep an eye on the weak riders and invite the strong riders to help. Communicate expectations and tell your clients what to expect. Don't ever lead people on a route that you have not done yourself if you can help it. Be honest about the terrain and what challenges the group may face.

The chances of your clients being more fit than you are slim. Don't judge a ride by how easy it is for you; make this adventure all about them and watch the excitement as they overcome challenges and learn a new sport. Remember that people are looking to discover something new and transformative from their experience with you. If you've planned a full day cycling fitness retreat, end with a celebratory dinner. These are always fun gatherings where the group can talk about the day—and plan the next adventure!

Plan your position on the ride

You'll want everyone to approach the ride with as much gusto and enthusiasm as you do, but do be patient. Some people are going to open it up and ride hard while others are there to socialize. Unless everyone in the group is exactly the same fitness and skill level, you can expect the group to quickly get spread out.

Trying to shepherd everyone safely during a ride can get very stressful. It's often not possible for you to keep an eye on every single rider, and you can wear yourself out fast by hanging with the front of the pack and turning around to chase the stragglers. If you're guiding alone (which I don't recommend), position yourself somewhere in the middle to front of the pack. You should be able to easily look ahead to the lead riders and behind you at those in the back of the pack. If there are two of you guiding, one of you will want to position yourself at the front of the pack with the strong riders while the other rides "sweep," keeping the riders in the rear within eyesight.

Don't forget the group photo. You want something the client can share with friends on social media that shows them what an amazing adventure they just had with you. Somewhere between handing out route notes and everyone collecting their bikes is usually the best time to take a picture of the group.

Review – Fitness Adventure Design

True/False

Select the answer that best fits the statement by circling true or false.

1. Fitness and skill level mean essentially the same thing when evaluating a client for appropriate activity intensity.

   a. True
   b. False

2. In general, once you know how to match the frequency, intensity, and time concepts to your clients' fitness levels, it will be easy to choose the type of activity.

   a. True
   b. False

3. It is a good idea to always do a pre-trip visit to a venue to test it out and inspect the area.

   a. True
   b. False

4. Intuition involves making decisions based on conscious reasoning.

   a. True
   b. False

5. A retreat where the clients participate in hiking to a lake and then stand up paddling for a set amount of time and then hiking back to the starting point would be considered a multi-sport retreat.

   a. True
   b. False

Multiple Choice

Circle the letter that corresponds to the correct answer for each question, below.

1. Which of the following apply to the T in FITT that stands for 'time?'

   a. Duration of the day as a whole
   b. Length of each individual activity
   c. Introducing the activity at the appropriate point in training
   d. All of the above

2. Exercises designed to improve the performance of everyday, real-life movements.

   a. Cluster exercises
   b. Functional exercises
   c. Intuitive exercises
   d. Frequency exercises

3. A successful trip is one that is carefully _____ with clear _____.

   a. Planned, timelines
   b. Copied, back-up plans
   c. Researched on the internet, links
   d. Marketed, revenue streams

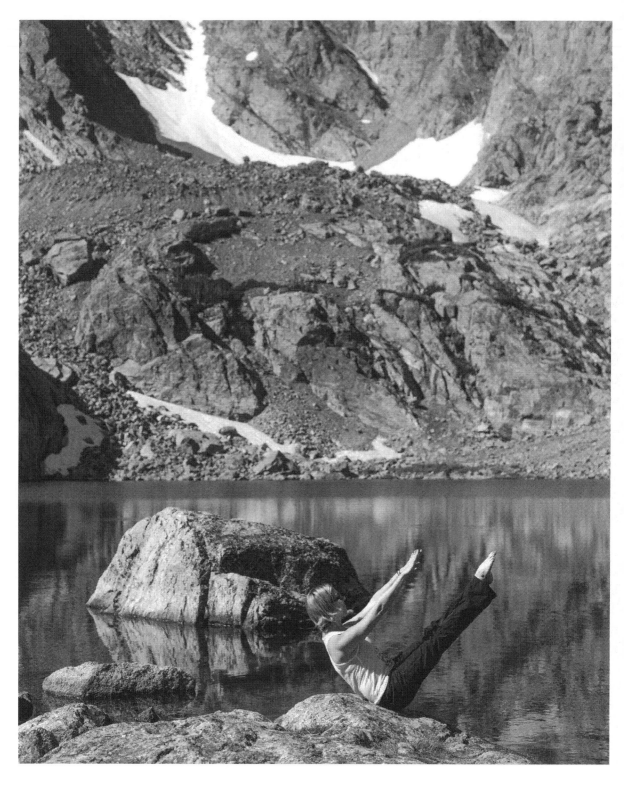

ADVENTURES IN MOTHER NATURE'S GYM

PART 6
THE SOL GUIDE METHOD
BODY-WEIGHT EXERCISE ARSENAL

"With a few exceptions, the great geniuses of history were gifted

with remarkable physical energy and aptitude, none more so

than [Leonardo] Da Vinci."

MICHAEL J. GELB

When I'm leading an outdoor fitness retreat I want the structured workout period to be very simple and relatively short, stripped of all but the most minimal of equipment – no music, no televisions, no cardio equipment, no mirrors… I think you get what I'm saying. If I can't teach a great core/functional workout that prepares someone for full-on activity using nothing but a yoga mat and their own body-weight, then perhaps I need to go back to the drawing board and start all over again. This is Mother Nature's Gym, after all!

The truth is that if you're a personal trainer coming from a traditional gym setting, or even a yoga instructor who teaches in a hot studio surrounded by three walls and, if you're lucky, a window, you may feel that training without the accoutrement of equipment and toys is a real challenge. Similarly, group exercise instructors may be wary of breaking from tradition and teaching more traditional strength training exercises.

Keep in mind that your client may feel vulnerable as well, stripped of the weights, machines, and classrooms full of people to hide beyond. Hopefully smart phones don't work in the outdoor location you've chosen – but even that could leave clients feeling more vulnerable and anxious. This is an opportunity for you (both) to be creative. Go back to the basics of everyday human movement to deliver an effective workout using nothing but the bare minimum. How did our ancient ancestors move before there was gym equipment?

The exercises presented in this chapter are designed to be a core/functional workout, performed using only body weight. There are endless possibilities to progress the exercises and workout sequences to more advanced and challenging levels, whether by increasing or decreasing the speed, number of sets and repetitions or range of motion, by interchanging specific exercises, or by using a few simple props (such as bands, suspension systems, etc.) that you can throw in your car or backpack.

Exercise Clusters

Each of the exercises in the Sol Guide Method 'exercise clusters' aids in increasing blood flow to major muscle groups, improves healthy biomechanics, and complements the movement patterns of each specific outdoor adventure (i.e. hiking, cycling, stand up paddling). Some exercises, like the breathing exercises and Qigong twists, for example, help relax people's nerves before trying something new and potentially unnerving, like stand up paddling on the water or road biking on challenging terrain through an unknown countryside. Others, like the plank and side lunge, featured below, are so foundational and beneficial that they can be used throughout all of the sport-specific sequences outlined.

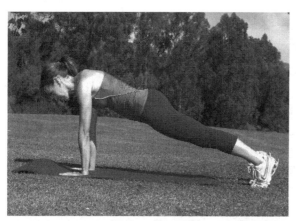

Examples

A plank is one example of a body-weight exercise with wide-ranging benefits to the body. The side lunge can be used for a variety of warm ups and cool downs and is a great way to introduce movement in the frontal plane.

Plank

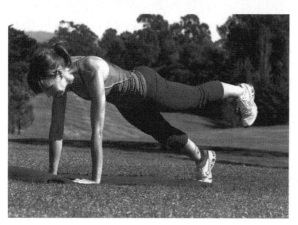

From a standing position, drop to all fours. Hands are directly under the shoulders. Extend the legs out behind you to balance on the toes. Eyes look down without dropping the head. The hips lift toward the sky, tilted slightly forward. Engage the pelvic floor. Hold.

Side Lunge

From standing, take a big step to one side. Sit back in the hips, keeping the chest lifted and eyes forward. Bend at the knees, but keep them well behind the toes. Push off of the outstretched leg to return to the start position. Complete one leg and then switch sides.

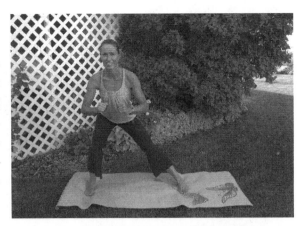

To do these exercises you need a flat surface—grass, sand, a wooden platform or pier work well. Even a cemented courtyard at a boutique hotel will work just fine as a warm up surface before a hike or bike ride. Yoga mats are optional but certainly preferred when lying on the ground.

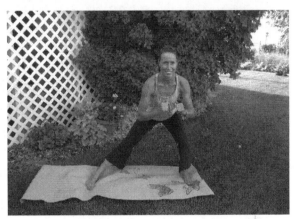

You can mix and match any of the exercises on the following pages to create a great outdoor workout that complements your outdoor adventure. I've grouped the clusters into a few different workouts that I like to use prior to leading my main outdoor adventures, which are hiking, biking, and stand up paddling. But you can just as easily swap out one cluster for a different one, or pair it with a variety of outdoor adventures. Play around with these and see what works for you - and definitely add your own favorite exercises to the mix!

- Dynamic Warm Up
- Breathing and Relaxation Sequence
- Stand Up Paddle and Water Sports Warm Up
- Hiking Exercise Sequence
- Cycling Exercise Sequence
- Mat-Based Core Workout

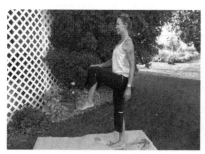 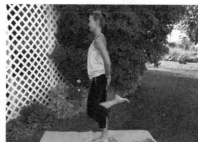 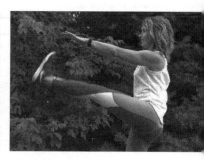

Dynamic Warm Up Sequence

This sequence is great for all age groups and fitness levels. Use it to enhance healthy movement patterns before activity, or as a cool down after the main event. Advanced athletes can perform these exercises at a rapid pace, like a track drill for runners. Here I demonstrate each movement slowly from a standing position.

You may notice that some of the exercise videos are used across several activities. This just goes to reinforce the idea that a given exercise can be interchanged and add value to a variety of recreational activities and movement objectives. Imagine, having a toolbox of very basic movements instead of machinery – what a relief!

High Knees

Stand with the feet directly under the hips. Knees slightly bent. Chest lifted and eyes straight ahead. Alternating legs, lift one leg off the ground, bringing the knee toward the opposite hand. Allow the weight to shift side to side while balancing on one leg. Repeat.

Butt Kickers

Stand with the feet slightly wider than the hips. Knees slightly bent. Chest lifted and eyes straight ahead. Alternating legs, bring the heel toward the butt, keeping the knee pointed directly toward the ground. Make a mental note of differences between each leg.

Straight Leg Kicks

Stand with the feet directly under the hips. Knees slightly bent. Chest and arms lifted and eyes straight ahead. Remaining straight at the knees, lift one leg forward, extending toward the hands. Alternate legs, keeping the chest lifted throughout the exercise. No rotation of the upper body.

Breathing and Relaxation Sequence

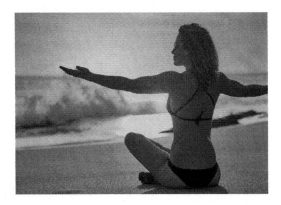

The breath is often used as the focus of meditation. Researchers have found that taking five deep breaths signals the parasympathetic nervous system to kick in, reducing the production of the stress hormone cortisol. Add an audible sigh on the exhale for the added bonus of the feel-good hormone oxytocin.

Use these deep breathing sequences to help your client become relaxed and focused. These are great to set the mood before the main activity or workout or as part of the cool down, especially if you're working with beginners who may feel a sense of anxiety about the adventure. Perform 10–20 repetitions of each exercise.

Side Stretch/Ribcage Opener
Stand with the feet wider than the hips. Knees slightly bent. Raise one arm out to the side and above the head as you take a big breath inward. As you exhale, drop to the opposite side, reaching toward the ground. Return to center and switch sides, settling into a slow, deep breathing pattern.

Cleansing Breath
Stand with the feet wider than the hips. Knees slightly bent. The arms reach downward and together, harnessing earth energy. Slowly take a deep breath in as the arms glide upward in front of the body. As the arms reach the face exhale, releasing energy toward the sky.

Energizing Breath
Stand with the feet wider than the hips. Knees slightly bent, hands over the heart. Slowly take a deep breath in as you open the arms out wide, turning the palms toward the sky. Pause. As you slowly exhale, return the hands to the heart.

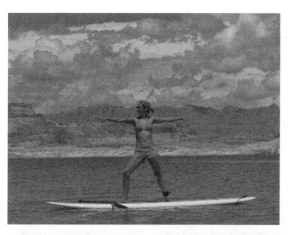

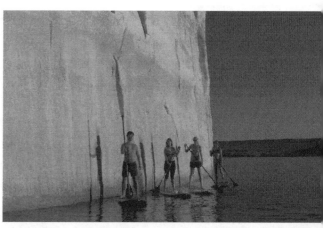

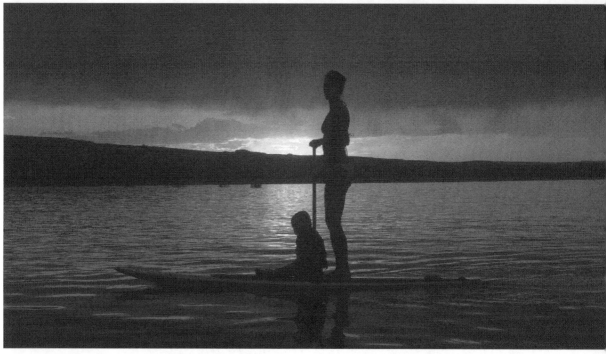

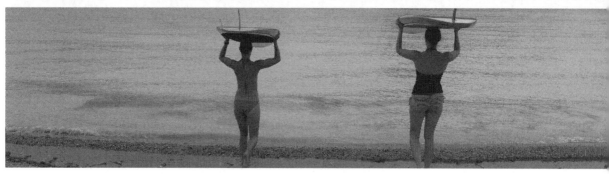

Stand Up Paddling

Before we jump in to the stand up paddle exercise sequence, let's talk a little about SUP. One of my favorite outdoor fitness retreat activities, SUP is unique because it offers something so out of the ordinary for a personal trainer and fitness instructor: a complete mind/body workout with the added mental bonus of being in close proximity to the water and aquatic life. There's something special about feeling like you're walking on water. You see things from a totally different perspective, settling into a low-impact rhythm and flow that's hard to find from other sports.

Ask anyone in the SUP industry and they'll be the first to tell you it's the fastest growing sport in the world. I stood on a board for the first time in 2008 and never looked back. I had to have one. Of course, one board turned into four or five, a few fantastic ambassador opportunities, and many more watermen and women friends along the way.

SUP is one of Sol Fitness Adventures foundational outdoor activities. I spent a weekend in Newport Beach getting my stand up paddle instructor certification and became the first person to be granted a commercial permit to guide SUP lessons in a U.S. National Park. You'll want to read Adventures in Mother Natures Gym: The Business Manual if guiding in a National Park is something you dream of doing – my learning curve will save you a lot of time in the long run!

Benefits of SUP

The workout you get from paddling is total body. From the ground – or board - up, every major muscle group is working. The legs might look passive, but there's actually quite a bit of isometric contraction happening through the major muscles of the legs and feet. Stabilizing muscles fire from the ankles through the knees and hips. Quads and hamstrings are engaged in a subtle dance of agonist/antagonist.

The more efficient you become with the paddle stroke, the more rotational torque you can get using your core. Chest, back and arms are in constant motion.

Stand up paddling is one of my favorite ways to improve balance and core strength. It's a fantastic way to spend time on the ocean for people who can't get the hang of surfing or hate getting pummeled by the waves when paddling out (I'm one of those people!). SUP can be done on a river, an inland lake, an estuary, or a bay. Teach a client to paddle once and chances are they'll do it again wherever they go in the world.

Have you been stand up paddling before? If so, what was your favorite SUP experience? If you haven't been stand up paddling, is there a water body near where you live that could you go to try it? If standing on water isn't your thing, what about kayaking or canoeing? How can you incorporate water into an outdoor fitness retreat for your clients?

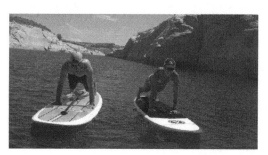

Stand Up Paddle and Water Sports Sequence

Water and paddling sports require coordinated movements of the upper and lower body in addition to rotational core movements. This standing sequence uses body weight only and is done at the water's edge as preparation for the paddle. You'll want to teach some sport-specific dry land training as well, but it all begins with preparing the body first.

This exercise sequence activates the large muscle groups of the lower body and core as well as the spine and shoulder stabilizers. Perform 2-3 sets, 12–20 repetitions of each exercise.

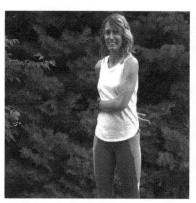 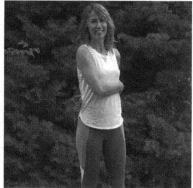

Qigong Kidney Taps

Stand with your feet slightly wider than the hips, knees slightly bent. Chest lifted and eyes straight ahead. Slowly begin to rotate the shoulders, allowing the arms to swing around the body. The back of the hands tap the lower back above the hips.

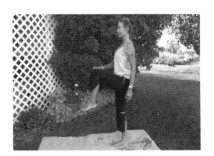

High knees

Stand with the feet directly under the hips. Knees slightly bent. Chest lifted and eyes straight ahead. Alternating legs, lift one leg off the ground, bringing the knee toward the opposite hand. Allow the weight to shift side to side while balancing on one leg. Repeat.

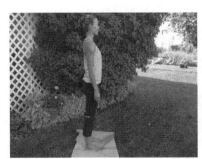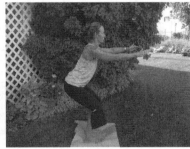

Squats

Stand with your feet slightly wider than the hips. Chest lifted and eyes straight ahead. Lift the toes slightly, shifting the weight to the heels. Moving from the hips first, sit your butt back, as if sitting in a chair. Keep the knees behind the toes. To stand bring the hips forward over the knees.

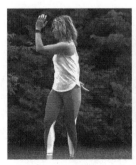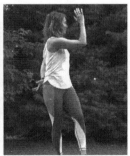

Brazilian Capoeira Twists

Stand with the feet slightly wider than the hips. Knees slightly bent. Chest lifted and eyes straight ahead. Alternating legs, kick forward into a toe tap, allowing the upper body to rotate toward the forward leg. Focus on engaging the abdominals as you rotate with purpose.

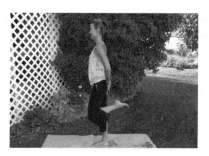

Butt Kickers

Stand with the feet slightly wider than the hips. Knees slightly bent. Chest lifted and eyes straight ahead. Alternating legs, bring the heel toward the butt, keeping the knee pointed directly toward the ground. Make a mental note of differences between each leg.

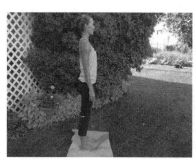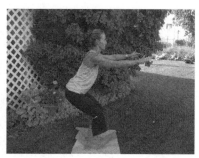

Quick Squats

Stand with your feet slightly wider than the hips. Chest lifted and eyes straight ahead. Lift the toes slightly, shifting the weight to the heels. Moving from the hips first, sit your butt back, as if sitting in a chair. Keep the knees behind the toes. Try to complete one squat per second.

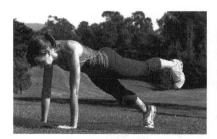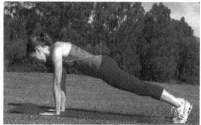

Plank with Alternating Leg Lift

From a standing position, drop to all fours on the hands and knees. Hands are directly under the shoulders. Extend the legs out behind you to balance on the toes. Eyes look down. The hips lift toward the sky, tilted slightly forward. Engage the pelvic floor. Keeping the hips squared and the leg straight, lift one heel toward the sky. Alternate.

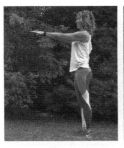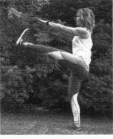

Straight leg kicks

Stand with the feet directly under the hips. Knees slightly bent. Chest and arms lifted and eyes straight ahead. Remaining straight at the knees, lift one leg forward, extending toward the hands. Alternate legs, keeping the chest lifted throughout the exercise. No rotation of the upper body.

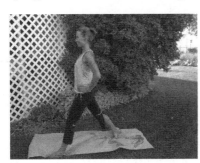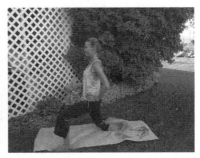

Standing lunge

From a standing position, step one leg forward, hip width apart. Keep the chest lifted and the eyes straight ahead. Bending the back knee, lower the hips toward the ground. Keep the front knee behind the toes. Drive the front heel into the ground as you lift the hips to return to standing.

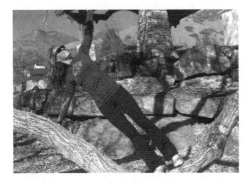

Side plank

Lie on your side along the back edge of your mat, all of the major joints inline. Place the elbow or hand directly under the shoulder as you raise the hips toward the sky. Lift until there's a straight line through the shoulders, hips, knees, and ankles. Raise the opposite arm toward the sky and hold.

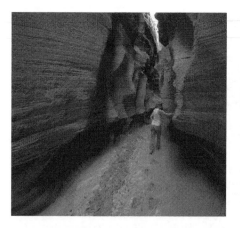
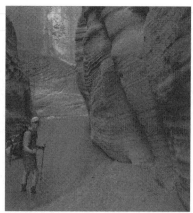
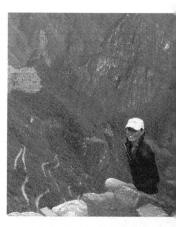
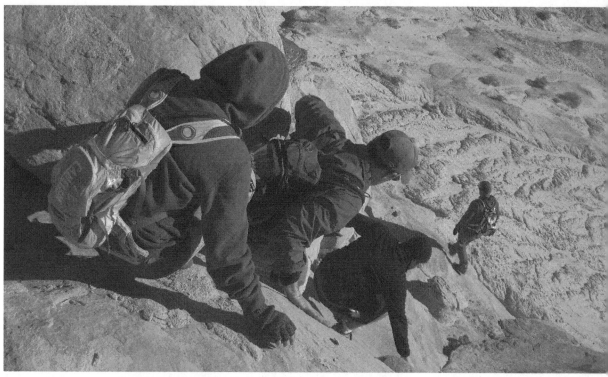
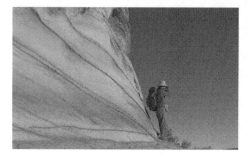
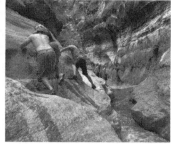
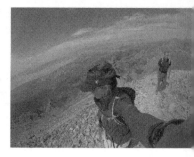

Hiking

There are many benefits to hiking. For one, it's easier on the body than running, which makes it a great choice for clients with knee pain (I'm one of those people now that I'm in my 40's). Most people can hike much farther than they can run, making it an incredible method of getting far into the backcountry and away from crowds, where you can really access the benefits of the great outdoors. Slowing down the pace creates the space to hear the sound of birds, watch the butterflies, and settle into a nice rhythmic movement pattern. You can select challenging trails that match the fitness level and specific goals of your clients or even use a hiking calorie calculator to get an idea of how many calories your hike will burn.

Hiking also offers physiological benefits. If you remember reading about the green mind earlier in the book (MW reference the chapter), you will recall that being in a forest calms the sympathetic nervous system, allowing the mind and body to restore itself and have a rest.

Most of my outdoor fitness retreats have centered around hiking, whether it's a short hike along the Lake Powell shoreline or a multi-day southern Utah National Park Trip. In 2008 I guided a challenging four-day backpacking trip through a slot canyon near Zion National Park. After a difficult hike out of the canyon my client turned to me and said, "next year, you're taking us to hike the Inca Trail to Machu Picchu Mel!" In 2009 we did just that.

My point in sharing my own stories and experiences is to invite you to pull out your bucket list and make it a reality. Don't wait til you retire or save enough money, plan a fitness retreat and make it happen! I promise you, if you have clients who love and trust you and know that you love to explore the outdoors, they're going to want to join your fitness retreats. If they're anything like my own clients, they'll do everything they can to help you spread the word and be successful.

JOURNAL ENTRY - HIKING

Think about a hike you have been on that was not only physically exhilarating, but also mentally stimulating. What was the experience like? If you haven't ever been on an epic hike, imagine what it would be like to explore your dream destination on foot. Put as much detail into your response as possible. This journal entry is only for you and may provide inspiration for future treks.

Hiking Exercise Sequence

The exercises in this sequence target the hips, lower legs, and core stabilizers. It's not necessary to push the legs to fatigue during a warm up. The legs are going to get plenty of exercise during the hike itself. But you do want to 'turn on' small stabilizing muscle groups around the joints. Firing the abdominals and spinal stabilizers will help integrate movements and provide a little extra support while carrying a backpack. The warm-up is especially helpful if it's a long hike and for people with back or joint problems.

Whether you're hiking, running, or speed walking, you can help your client prepare for the activity with the simple exercises in this sequence. These exercises warm up the major muscle groups in the lower body and core.

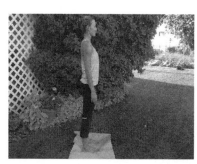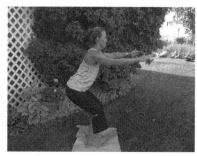

Squats

Stand with your feet slightly wider than the hips. Chest lifted and eyes straight ahead. Lift the toes slightly, shifting the weight to the heels. Moving from the hips first, sit your butt back, as if sitting in a chair. Keep the knees behind the toes. To stand bring the hips forward over the knees.

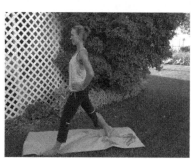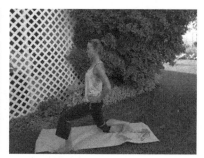

Standing Lunges

From a standing position, step one leg forward, hip width apart. Keep the chest lifted and the eyes straight ahead. Bending the back knee, lower the hips toward the ground. Keep the front knee behind the toes. Drive the front heel into the ground as you lift the hips to return to standing.

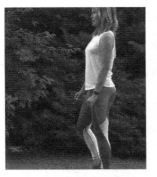 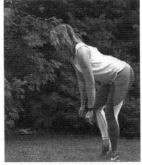

Single Leg Dead Left

From standing, shift weight to one leg, keeping the other leg nearby for balance. Bend the standing knee slightly. Moving from the hips, hinge the upper body forward, keeping the spine straight, the eyes lifted. Return to start position and repeat.

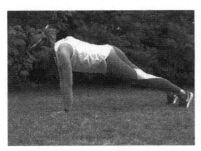 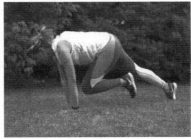

Plank Mountain Climber

Start on all fours, hands directly under the shoulders and legs extended behind you. The hips lift toward the sky, tilted slightly under. Draw one knee into the chest, tucking the pelvis and keeping the toes off the ground. Return to the start position and alternate.

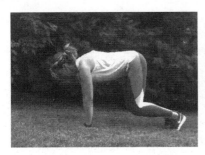 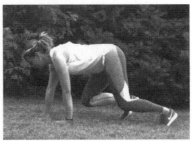

Bear Crawl

Start on all fours in a crouch position. Keeping the mid-section close to the ground, begin to travel forward by reaching out with the opposite arm and leg moving at the same time. Keep the body weight supported by the hands and feet until you reach your destination.

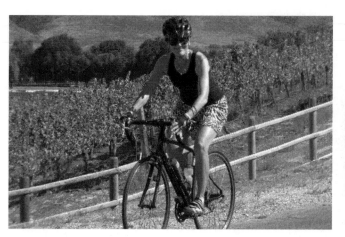

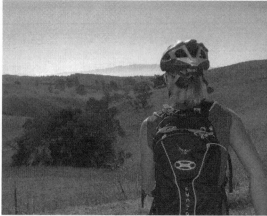

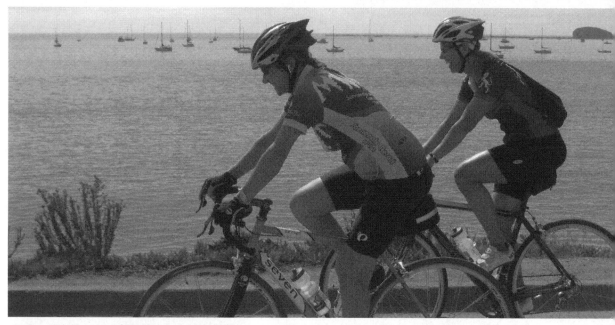

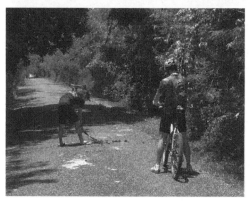

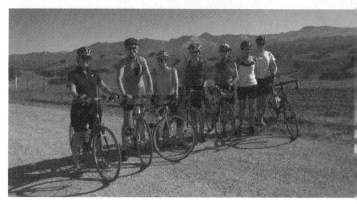

Cycling

Cycling . . . Now there's a sport for you! Have you ever heard the term suffer-fest? Serious cyclists seam to take pleasure in the pain of a punishing group ride. If you're a spin instructor reading this book you have endless opportunities to take your practice outdoors and lead exciting, even spectacular cycling trips!

Both road and mountain biking have been staples of Sol's outdoor fitness retreat offerings for years. One of my favorite trips involved a group of eight women from Colorado, each over the age of 55. We planned a six-day road biking fitness retreat through the vineyards of the Central Coast of California. One of the women was 70 years old and had never ridden a bike outside before. She wanted to come on the trip so badly that she trained in a spin studio for three months before the trip. The first day's ride hadn't even finished and she was already talking about next year's trip. It was a blast!

There are a lot of operational nuances to guiding a great cycling trip, but there isn't a cycling guide permit or license that I'm aware of. If you don't have time for a temp job guiding cycling trips, join forces with a tour operator who specializes in an area you want to explore and let them do all the dirty work. Then, just show up with your clients and have fun!

Chances are that your clients have always wanted to take a cycling trip. Don't help them prepare, only to send them off to an exotic location with a tour company like I did for several years – study this book and The Business Manual and you will be able to lead the trip yourself!

JOURNAL ENTRY - CYCLING

Are you and your clients more likely to ride road bikes along a scenic coastline or mountain bikes on a winding single track trail through the woods or Moab's slickrock? Perhaps e-biking through the Emmental Valley of Switzerland to a cheese factory sounds more intriguing (actually it is – I did that on one trip!). In either case, I recommend a bit of core exercise before you jump on the bikes, and certainly a great stretch or yoga session after the ride.
What type of exercises do you think would be good to warm up for a cycling trip? To get you started I'll share Sol's comprehensive cycling warm up sequence next.

Cycling Exercise Sequence

This sequence is a combination of grounding exercises that target the hips and legs as well as core stabilizers that support strong cycling. I've used some very basic movements that you'll recognize and included one move called the 'Founder,' from a method called Foundation which was created to support healthy backs. These exercises have proven effective for everyone from professional athletes to desk jockeys with back pain.

Use these exercises as a warm up before cycling. The exercises primarily target the large muscle groups of the lower body while engaging the abdominal muscles and lower back for added stability and to take pressure off of the hips and shoulders. Perform 2-3 sets, 12–15 repetitions of each movement.

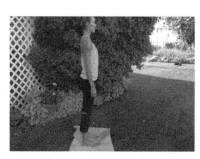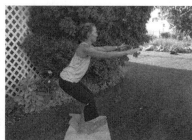

Squats

Stand with your feet slightly wider than the hips. Chest lifted and eyes straight ahead. Lift the toes slightly, shifting the weight to the heels. Moving from the hips first, sit your butt back, as if sitting in a chair. Keep the knees behind the toes. To stand bring the hips forward over the knees.

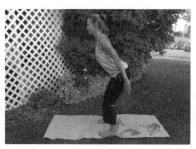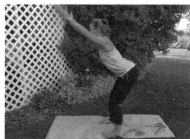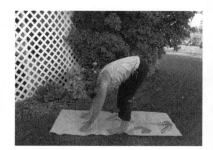

Founder

With feet under the hips, lift the toes and shift the weight into the heels, reaching back with the arms. Lean way back at the hips, keeping the spine straight. Arms reach overhead. Slowly hinge forward from the hips and allow the upper body to "ragdoll" as you relax. Keep the knees slightly bent as you move from the hips to return to start position.

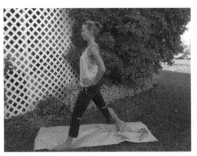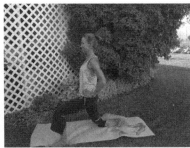

Standing Lunge

From a standing position, step one leg forward, hip width apart. Keep the chest lifted and the eyes straight ahead. Bending the back knee, lower the hips toward the ground. Keep the front knee behind the toes. Drive the front heel into the ground as you lift the hips to return to standing.

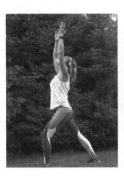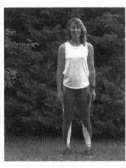

Standing Hip Flexor Stretch

From a standing position take a big step back, keeping the feet hip-width apart. Lift the toes in the front leg, knee slightly bent. Raise the arms overhead and look back as you hinge backward from the hips. Lean the upper body in the direction of the forward leg. Slowly return to start.

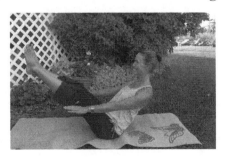

Boat Pose

From a seated position, rock back onto the tailbone, lifting the hands and legs away from the ground. Imagine creating the shape of the letter V out of your body. Keep the chest lifted. Knees can remain slightly bent or straight behind the knee.

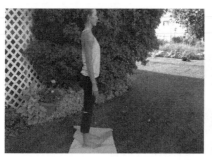 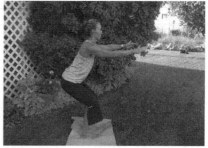

Quick Squat

Stand with your feet slightly wider than the hips. Chest lifted and eyes straight ahead. Lift the toes slightly, shifting the weight to the heels. Moving from the hips first, sit your butt back, as if sitting in a chair. Keep the knees behind the toes. Try to complete one squat per second.

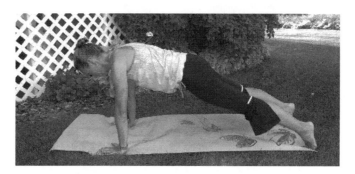

Mat-Based Core Workout

The core workout is designed to be a complete workout and may take 45 minutes to an hour to complete, depending on the number of sets and reps you choose to do. Use the core workout as preparation for the major outdoor activity or as a stand-alone workout during a full day outdoor fitness retreat. The core series can be taught as we've shown here, without any props. For a more athletic or challenging workout, add props like medicine balls, Pilates® circles, hand weights, and Glider discs.

You should recognize most of these exercises. These are the good old standbys - combinations of functional, rehab, and core exercises as well as Pilates®, and yoga disciplines.

All you need for this complete core workout is a mat or towel and a flat space. I've done this workout on wooden decks, grass, even concrete platforms with extra thick mats. Perform 2-3 sets, 12–15 repetitions of each exercise.

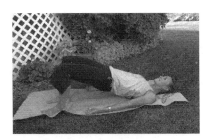

Bridges

Lie flat on your back, arms at the side and palms facing upward. Knees are bent with the feet parallel. Engage the pelvic floor. Press both feet into the ground, keeping contact with the entire foot, as you press the hips toward the sky. Form a straight line from the shoulder, hips and knees.

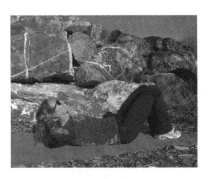

Ceiling Crunch

Lie flat on your back, knees bent and feet parallel. Keeping the elbows wide, allow the fingers to gently support the head. Engage the pelvic floor. Imagine a string attached at your sternum gently lifting you toward the sky without curling the spine forward.

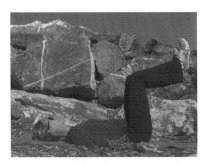

Reverse Crunch

Lie flat on your back, arms resting at your sides with the palms turned upward. Bring the knees toward the chest, keeping a 90-degree bend at the hips, knees, and ankles. Engage the pelvic floor as you slowly curl the tailbone off of the ground, bringing the knees toward the face.

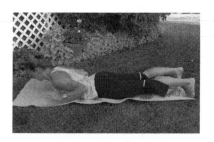

Back Extension

Lie flat on your stomach with the legs extended. Activate posterior muscles by flexing the toes, pushing the backs of the knees toward the sky and raising the chest slightly away from the ground. Arms are bent at your sides, shoulder blades engaged. Lift the upper body off of the ground.

Quadruped Extension

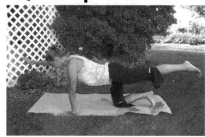

Start on all fours, hands directly under the shoulders, knees under the hips. Engage the pelvic floor muscles as you square the hips. Keeping the eyes downward, slowly reach one arm forward at the same time you extend the opposite leg behind you, pressing the heel and extending behind the knee.

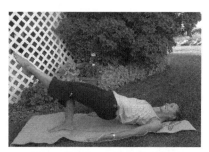

Single Leg Bridges

Lie flat on your back, arms to the side with the palms facing upward. Knees are bent with the feet parallel. Extend one leg straight toward the sky, remaining connected at the knees. Press the grounded foot into the earth, sending the hips, squared, up to the sky.

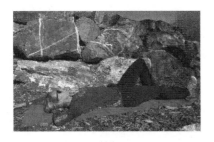
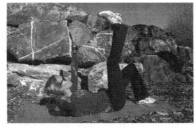

Opposite Arm and Leg Crunch

Lie flat on your back with one knee bent, the opposite arm gently supporting the head. Opposite arm and leg are extended, flat on the ground. Slowly raise the opposite arm and leg as you lift your chest toward the sky, keeping the shoulders squared.

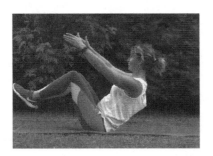
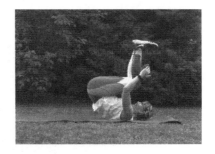

Pilates® Rolling Like a Ball

Start from a seated position. Bend the knees, bringing them toward the chest as you hold gently behind the knees. Round the spine as you rock backward and roll onto the upper back. Control the momentum as you roll forward, pausing slightly at the start position before repeating.

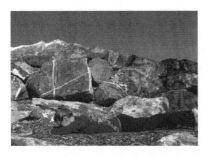
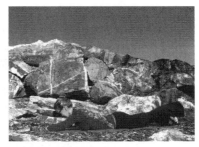

Pilates® Swimmers

Lie on your stomach with arms and legs extended. Point the toes and engage the pelvic floor as you raise the arms, legs, and chest off the ground. Lift the eyes and the opposite arm and leg away from the ground, alternating in a swimming motion.

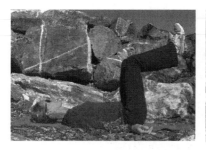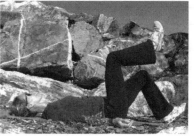

Pilates® Leg Drops

Lie flat on your back, arms at your sides with the palms facing upward. Bring the knees toward the chest, keeping a 90-degree bend at the hips, knees, and ankles. Keeping the hips squared and the joints at 90 degrees, slowly lower one leg toward the ground, alternating.

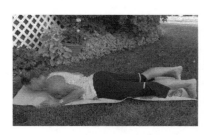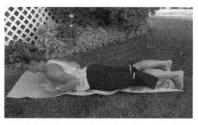

Wide Leg Back Extension

Lie flat on your stomach with the legs extended wider than the mat. Activate posterior muscles by flexing the toes, pushing the backs of the knees toward the sky and raising the chest slightly away from the ground. Arms are bent at your sides, shoulder blades engaged. Lift the upper body off of the ground.

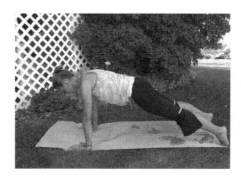

Wide Leg Plank

From all fours, place hands directly under the shoulders. Extend the legs wider than the mat and balance on the toes. Eyes look down without dropping the head. The hips lift toward the sky, tilted slightly forward. Engage the pelvic floor. Hold.

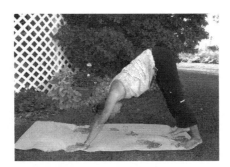

Downward Facing Dog

From all fours, send the hips up toward the sky, allowing the heels to drop to the ground. Draw the knees up toward the hips as you tuck the pelvis slightly toward the chest. Eyes look up at the belly as the arms push the spine away from the ground. Breathe.

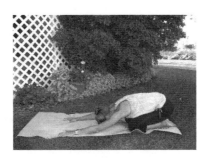

Child's Pose

From all fours, allow the body to come to a complete rest by sitting back on the heels. Bring the knees apart. Arms can remain forward or relaxed at your sides. Breathe deep and relax.

Online Video Library

I'm thrilled to offer my readers exclusive, complimentary access to the Body-Weight Exercise Arsenal Video Library. Visit Sol Fitness Adventures online to incorporate these exercises into your own outdoor fitness retreats. You'll find the library at: http://solfitnessadventures.com/mother-na-tures-gym-exercise-arsenal/

Program Review

Test your knowledge with a review of Adventures in Mother Nature's Gym. Though you won't be graded, it is a good idea to go back and retake review exercises throughout the book to study for the exam. Let these questions be a guide as you begin creating your own style of outdoor fitness retreats.

1. According to researcher Mihaly Csikszentmihaly, there are two required states of mind to enter the flow state. Which are they?

    a. Control and expertise
    b. Arousal and control
    c. Expertise and fear
    d. Fear and arousal

2. Basic responsibilities of an outdoor fitness guide include which of the following?

    a. Logistics
    b. Gear list and inspection
    c. Interpretation
    d. All of the above

3. When conducting a gear inspection prior to running a fitness retreat, red flags to look out for include which of the following?

    a. Brand new equipment
    b. Damaged equipment
    c. Competitor's brands
    d. Light reflecting properties

4. Checking local _____ refers to investigating what the weather, roads, and trails will look like during the time of your fitness retreat.

    a. Logistics
    b. Opinions
    c. Experts
    d. Conditions

5. The first step if someone is injured is to do what?

    a. Call emergency contact
    b. Call the local authorities and 9-1-1
    c. Assess the situation and whether anyone else is in danger
    d. Deliver care until the authorities or EMS arrives

6. Common topics on a fitness retreat to consider preparing interpretive notes for include which of the following?

    a. What makes the people of the place unique
    b. Unique cultural practices
    c. Language translation
    d. Both a and b

7. Common logistical elements a guide is responsible for during a fitness retreat include which of the following?

    a. Start and end locations
    b. Making hotel reservations for the guest
    c. Purchasing required gear for the client
    d. Client hygiene

8. School-aged children require anywhere from _____ calories per day.

    a. 1,500 – 2,000
    b. 2,000 – 2,500
    c. 1,600 – 2,200
    d. 2,200 – 3,000

9. Major threats to wellness that the Sol Guide Method addresses include which of the following ailments?

    a. Digital distraction
    b. Sedentary lifestyle
    c. Nature deficit disorder
    d. All of the above

10. The minimum level of first aid training required to guide an outdoor fitness retreat is what?

    a. Adult First Aid and CPR
    b. Wilderness First Responder
    c. Wilderness First Aid
    d. Wilderness EMT

11. Main aspects of Program Design include which of the following?

    a. How to assess client needs and abilities
    b. How to choose the proper activities for a client
    c. How to program warm-ups and cool-down activities
    d. All of the above

12. Special populations that may require additional attention to detail during a fitness adventure include

    a. Teenagers
    b. Pregnant women
    c. Children
    d. Both b and c

13. Topics to consider while developing a safety talk include which of the following?

    a. How long is the activity?
    b. What factors are outside of my control?
    c. What factors pose the greatest risk to my clients?
    d. All of the above

14. The use of single words to illicit a relaxation and sensory response is called guided _____.

    a. Zen
    b. Creation
    c. Imagery
    d. Cueing

15. Intuitive training refers to using one's feelings to guide the decision making process

    a. True
    b. False

16. The FITT principles of program design include

    a. Time
    b. Therapy
    c. Functional
    d. Torque

17. Wellness travelers take trips with the specific intention of engaging in activities that maintain or improve their quality of life.

    a. True
    b. False

18. Creating accurate route notes requires

    a. The latest Google Map view of the area
    b. A GPS unit
    c. Exploring the route during pre-trip work
    d. Purchasing a software program from the local outdoor store

19. When guiding an outdoor fitness adventure it is best to always require that your clients do not drink alcohol

    a. True
    b. False

20. After you've mastered the concepts in Adventures in Mother Nature's Gym you will be qualified to call yourself a healer.

    a. True
    b. False

21. The best time to perform stretching or yoga exercises is at the _____ of the workout.

    a. Beginning
    b. End
    c. Rest phase
    d. Top

22. Beneficial electrolyte recovery drinks include

    a. Beer
    b. Coke
    c. Water
    d. Both a and c

23. Being _____ with the proper clothing, footwear, gear, and hydration is critical for optimum physical performance and your safety.

    a. Progressive
    b. Prepared
    c. Frugal
    d. Both a and c

24. The over-dependence on digital devices is called digital _____.

    a. Addiction
    b. Dependence
    c. Sociality
    d. Distraction

25. Wallace J. Nichols is one of the leading researchers in the theories of Red Mind.

    a. True
    b. False

26. To keep clients hydrated throughout the day encourage them to drink water at least every

    a. 10-minutes
    b. Hour
    c. Morning and night
    d. 20-minutes

27. The earth's magnetic frequency measures 7.83 Hz. What is this frequency called?

    a. Schumann resonance
    b. Einstein's theory of relativity
    c. Heinrich Hertz wave
    d. Red Mind

28. One of the countries leading the way in developing forest walking paths is which of the following?

    a. Argentina
    b. England
    c. Japan
    d. United States of America

29. Select the activity that will best allow the body to access the physiological responses described by Blue Mind:

    a. Walking in a forest
    b. Hiking in the desert
    c. Mountain biking
    d. Kayaking

30. Important categories to include on a gear list include which of the following?

    a. Digital devices
    b. Sun protection
    c. Clothing and shoes
    d. Both b and c

31. Swimming can create a brain response similar to that found during which activity?

    a. Meditation
    b. Studying
    c. Exercising
    d. Yoga

32. Extensive scientific evidence exists to support the theory of Red Mind.

    a. True
    b. False

33. The emotions associated with the Sol Guide Method concept of Red Mind include which of the following?

    a. Anger
    b. Type A personalities
    c. Anxiousness
    d. Love

34. The phrase Mother Nature's Gym refers to which of the following?

    a. The woo-woo spas along California's coastline
    b. The natural surroundings where fitness retreats take place
    c. City parks used to host boot camps
    d. Indoor/outdoor gyms

35. The ultimate objective of neuro-conservation is to accomplish which of the following?

    a. Influence public health for the better
    b. Drive votes to the Democratic party
    c. Save the planet
    d. Educate the general public on wildlife conservation

36. A pregnant client in her third trimester requires approximately how many calories per day?

    a. 2,000
    b. 1,500
    c. 3,000
    d. 2,400

37. Children are especially _____ to extremes in temperature.

    a. Resistant
    b. Responsive
    c. Resigned
    d. Susceptible

38. Overuse of electronic media has been shown to have which of the following impacts on human health?

    a. Improved concentration
    b. Reduced stress levels
    c. Decreased concentration
    d. Rich personal relationships

39. Blue Mind refers to which of the following responses of the human body/mind?

    a. Feelings of depression that settle in after leaving the ocean
    b. Feelings of joy and happiness that result from proximity to water
    c. Feelings of longing associated with water sports
    d. Open water swimmers

40. The effects of nature deficit disorder in children include which of the following?

    a. Fear of natural elements
    b. Attention disorders
    c. Depression
    d. Both b and c

41. The stress hormone _____ regulates function of the arteries.

    a. Dopamine
    b. Seratonin
    c. Endorphin
    d. Catecholamine

42. Cognitive reserve describes which characteristic of the brain?

    a. Ability to process new information
    b. Resilience to damage
    c. Regulation of physical movement
    d. Recollection of early memories

43. Benefits of aquatic exercise include which of the following?

    a. Balancing the stress hormone catecholamine
    b. Decreasing systolic blood pressure
    c. Providing the greatest amount of cognitive reserve
    d. Both a and c

44. A 2012 study measured the author's systolic blood pressure as _____ points higher than normal after walking in an urban environment, compared to _____ points lower than normal in the forest.

    a. 6; 6
    b. 10; 10
    c. 5; 10
    d. 10; 5

45. What is the maximum amount of time a beginner should spend doing a specific outdoor activity on their first outing?

    a. 60-minutes
    b. 30-minutes
    c. 90-minutes
    d. 120-minutes

46. The Center for Disease Control (CDC) ranked unipolar depression as the third most prevalent cause of disease burden worldwide in 2004.

    a. True
    b. False

47. Cerebral spinal centers containing life energy are called _____ in Indian Sanskrit.

    a. OM
    b. Frequencies
    c. Chakras
    d. Rishis

48. The 'fight or flight' response is regulated by which of the body's systems?

    a. Parasympathetic nervous system
    b. Adrenal-pituitary axis
    c. Autonomic nervous system
    d. Sympathetic nervous system

49. The phrase that describes the physiological responses of the human body/mind in outdoor green settings is termed _____.

    a. The Nature Cure
    b. Mother Nature's Gym
    c. Green Mind
    d. Forest Walking

50. The use of phrases that stimulate memory to illicit a relaxation response is called guided _____.

    a. Imagery
    b. Meditation
    c. Visualization
    d. Stimulation

51. _____ is defined as a feeling of reverential respect mixed with fear or wonder.

    a. Excitement
    b. Stoke
    c. Bliss
    d. Awe

52. Playing outside has been shown to provide which of the following health benefits in children?

    a. Fewer cavities
    b. Greater growth spurts
    c. Improved symptoms of ADHD
    d. Stronger bones

53. The emotional response of awe occurs when which of the following conditions exist?

    a. Fearing repercussions for one's actions
    b. Encountering an unexpected stimulus
    c. Anticipating a romantic encounter
    d. Making a mistake

54. Components of a trip that distinguish adventure travel from leisure travel include which of the following?

    a. Active physical participation
    b. Sleeping in the best hotels
    c. Paying the most for service
    d. Using a travel agent to make arrangements

55. According to the Center for Disease Control (CDC), post-traumatic stress disorder (PTSD) and phobias are categorized as which type of mental health disorder?

    a. Depression
    b. Personality disorders
    c. Anxiety disorders
    d. Both a and b

56. Reasons for making a pre-trip visit to the location of your fitness retreat include which of the following?

    a. Familiarizing yourself with the route
    b. Being aware of current conditions
    c. Building relationships with local service providers
    d. All of the above

57. When designing a fitness retreat using the exercises presented in this book, you have to follow the sequencing as precisely as taught.

    a. True
    b. False

58. _____ is defined as an exciting activity calling for enterprise and enthusiasm.

    a. Adventure
    b. Fitness
    c. Sol Guide Method
    d. Exercise

59. Author Melanie Webb gained her qualifications for developing the Sol Guide Method by working primarily in which two professions?

    a. Yoga and environmental consulting
    b. Personal training and wildlife biology
    c. Business and marketing
    d. Hospitality and tourism

60. New opportunities that will open to you once you begin planning your own outdoor fitness retreats include which of the following?

    a. Expanding your office to include the outdoors
    b. Diversifying income streams
    c. Adding skill sets to your professional toolbox
    d. All of the above

61. Completing your study of the Sol Guide Method will qualify you to design and lead fitness retreats under your own label.

    a. True
    b. False

62. Completing this book will enable you to run trips under the Sol Fitness Adventures label.

    a. True
    b. False

63. Bodyweight in excess of biological needs is defined as

    a. Morbidity
    b. Obesity
    c. Laziness
    d. Common

64. All drugs taken in excess have in common the direct activation of the brains' _____ system.

    a. Alarm
    b. Memory
    c. Reward
    d. Learning

65. The continual use of digital devices can elicit an _____ response in the brain.

    a. Alarm
    b. Addiction
    c. Relaxed
    d. Overuse

66. Qualities of being self-aware include

    a. Confidence
    b. Anxious
    c. Ability
    d. Both a and c

67. Way-shower, teacher, leader, and exemplar are all synonyms of which of the following roles?

    a. Guide
    b. Politician
    c. Judge
    d. Actress

68. The guide's motto is to "lead, _____, and help."

    a. Discipline
    b. Push
    c. Assist
    d. Prove

69. "Honor the gift of _____ your clients give you and you are bound to succeed as a guide."

    a. Gratitude
    b. Money
    c. Testimonials
    d. Trust

70. To be a good guide you must

    a. Know your limits
    b. Push your clients to their full capacity
    c. Always be in front of the group
    d. Have more certifications than the competition

71. As a guide you want to assist clients as they transfer skills mastered in the gym to physical _____ in an unfamiliar outdoor environment.

    a. Contests
    b. Challenges
    c. Discomfort
    d. Proficiency

72. The term flexibility, as used in the Sol Guide Method to define guide qualifications, means

    a. Full range of motion about a joint
    b. Being willing to give away your power
    c. The ability to adapt to unexpected situations
    d. Asking for group consensus in dangerous conditions

73. The term 'reconnection,' as it is used in this book, refers to helping people experience the instinctive mindset of which of the following concepts?

    a. Living in close relation to the Earth
    b. Wandering aimlessly
    c. Living with a tribe
    d. Connecting with supernatural energies

74. The role of the 'strong second' guide is to do what?

    a. Bring up the rear on outdoor activities
    b. Make all rental reservations
    c. Be physically stronger than the lead guide
    d. Assist the lead guide

75. Your most important work as a guide is to lead others to a _____ between themselves and the outdoors.

    a. Experience
    b. Challenge
    c. Reconnection
    d. Confrontation

76. Ways to reconnect with the Earth include

    a. Look up your location on Google Maps
    b. Pay money to your environmental activist group of choice
    c. Watch a sunrise or sunset
    d. Watch a nature program on television

77. 'Free play' is _____ time outside to play in the dirt, collect bugs, and be a kid.

    a. Structured
    b. Supervised
    c. Unstructured
    d. Endless

78. "_____ is voluntary, it's pleasurable, and it offers a sense of engagement."

    a. Running
    b. Play
    c. Working out
    d. Guiding

79. The purpose of performing a relaxation and breathing sequence prior to an outdoor activity is what?

    a. To help the client become relaxed and focused (correct)
    b. To create a spiritual climate for the client
    c. Teach your client the proper way to breathe
    d. Reminding the client of your expertise

80. It is critical that the dynamic warm up sequence be performed at slow speeds with little impact or vertical gain.

    a. True
    b. False

81. The three exercises that comprise the dynamic warm up include which of the following combinations?

    a. Squats, planks, lunges
    b. Bear crawl, plank mountain climbers, straight leg kicks
    c. High knees, butt-kickers, straight let kicks
    d. Qigong twists, capoeira twists, full body rotation

82. When guiding the client through the breathing and relaxation exercises it is very important to remind them to keep the knees in what position?

    a. Locked
    b. Behind the toes
    c. Engaged
    d. Slightly bent

83. Stand up paddling is a _____ body workout.

    a. Upper
    b. Lower
    c. Middle
    d. Total

84. What is the primary purpose(s) for leading the body-weight exercise clusters prior to performing the outdoor activity?

    a. Enhance healthy biomechanics
    b. Attract the attention of passersby
    c. Increase blood flow to major muscle groups
    d. Both a and c

85. The Sol Guide Method exercise clusters can easily be _____ and _____ by adding props and gear.

    a. Simplified
    b. Progressed
    c. Adjusted
    d. Both b and c

86. The best time to perform the core workout is _____ the outdoor activity.

    a. During
    b. After
    c. Before
    d. Throughout

87. Stand up paddling primarily requires which two types of movement?

    a. Rotation and isometrics
    b. Fast twitch, coordinated
    c. Balance and rotation
    d. Slow twitch, rotation

88. Being in a forest calms the _____ nervous system.

    a. Parasympathetic
    b. Sympathetic
    c. Autonomic
    d. Both a and c

89. Guiding a road cycling fitness retreat requires a sport-specific certification.

    a. True
    b. False

90. When training someone using only body weight, one way to increase difficulty is to increase which of the following variables?

    a. Speed of movement
    b. Number of repetitions
    c. The volume in your voice
    d. Both a and b

91. To perform the exercises presented in the Sol Guide Method exercise clusters, you must have which of the following?

    a. A mat or towel
    b. A bag of gym props
    c. Pilates balls and circles
    d. A clipboard

92. The core exercise cluster taught in the Sol Guide Method is adapted from which mind/body disciplines?

    a. Floor Pilates
    b. Yoga
    c. Cross-fit
    d. Both a and b

93. Of the following commonly used disciplines and principles, which best describes the method of program design used to plan the exercise components of a fitness retreat?

    a. FITT
    b. HIT
    c. MAT
    d. None of the above

94. The higher the precision of movement required for the outdoor activity during your fitness retreat, the more emphasis you'll place on _____ rather than _____.

    a. Mobility; balance
    b. Skill; fitness
    c. Strength; mobility
    d. Fitness; skill

95. The goal is to design activities to _____ client's capabilities, not _____ them.

    a. Highlight; diminish
    b. Develop; ignore
    c. Train; overtrain
    d. Challenge; overlook

96. Leading a client on an outdoor fitness retreat requires that you design the program to take into account fitness level and _____.

    a. Maturity
    b. Gender
    c. Competition
    d. Terrain

97. Which training principle(s) will influence the ability of a client to learn the skills of a new outdoor sport?

    a. Specificity
    b. Time
    c. Intensity
    d. All of the above

98. In addition to studying this book and the Sol Guide Method, a sport-specific certification may be required to lead which type of outdoor activities?

　　a. Road cycling
　　b. Technical sports such as rock climbing or skiing
　　c. Water-based activities including swimming
　　d. Both b and c

99. The outdoors is full of _____ forces.

　　a. Predictable
　　b. Uncontrollable
　　c. Unknown
　　d. Spiritual

100. On an outdoor trip you can expect the _____.

　　a. Usual
　　b. Best
　　c. Worst
　　d. Unexpected

101. _____ is a primary concern when guiding older adults on outdoor fitness retreats.

　　a. Hearing
　　b. Vision
　　c. Memory
　　d. Mobility

Program Review: Answers

Check your answers to the program review against the answers below.

1. b	21. b	41. d	61. a	81. c
2. d	22. d	42. b	62. b	82. d
3. b	23. b	43. d	63. b	83. d
4. d	24. d	44. a	64. c	84. d
5. c	25. b	45. c	65. b	85. d
6. d	26. d	46. a	66. d	86. c
7. a	27. a	47. c	67. a	87. c
8. c	28. c	48. d	68. c	88. b
9. d	29. d	49. c	69. d	89. b
10. c	30. d	50. c	70. a	90. d
11. d	31. a	51. d	71. b	91. a
12. d	32. b	52. c	72. c	92. d
13. d	33. d	53. b	73. a	93. a
14. c	34. b	54. a	74. d	94. b
15. a	35. a	55. c	75. c	95. a
16. a	36. d	56. d	76. c	96. d
17. a	37. d	57. b	77. c	97. d
18. c	38. c	58. a	78. b	98. d
19. b	39. b	59. b	79. a	99. b
20. b	40. d	60. d	80. b	100. d
				101. d

ACKNOWLEDGEMENTS

After all the ups and downs of entrepreneur life I never would have imagined that the act of sitting down to write a book about what I've learned guiding outdoor fitness retreats would have gone so smoothly. My colleague Sara Anisman first suggested the idea, and I knew in that moment that I had to find a way to get it done. Finding the right avenue to publish and take these concepts to the world, however, took a bit of trial, error, and even failure. The first edition, an online interactive course entitled *Sol Guide*, was accessible for less than a year. Now that the book is published I'm so thrilled to assist my peers in the fitness, recreation, and healthcare industries as you take the leap to leave the indoor settings and lead more people into an active outdoor lifestyle.

In love and respect to the following individuals who have supported me in this journey:

The Creatives: Monica and Dan Ervin, Aaron Gaitan, Brian Bunton, Pete Iccabazzi, Ryan Richardson, Jacqueline Sweet and Anton Hafele.

Family, friends, and mentors: My parents Merrill and Lynnette Webb, who made sports and nature a significant part of my upbringing; my sisters and brother April, Lindy, and Tyler for supporting my entrepreneurial inclinations from a young age; my niece Sadie Williams Hoyt for her expert final editing skills; Barbara Crane-Gilbert, Amie Kane-Lee, Yermo and Anne-Francoise Welsh, Cari Gray, Daniel Dayton, Barb, Jennifer, and Hamilton Easter for the encouragement, mentoring, and enduring friendship; Kathy Smith, whose expert insight was critical as I weighed my decision to jump in and make my contribution; the many colleagues I've worked with and learned from and who inspire me to be my best, from The Sports Club/LA in Washington, D.C. to Snowcreek Athletic Club and Montecito Country Club in California, Amangiri and Waldorf Astoria Park City in Utah.

The Creator, for the gifts and wonders of the human body and for a lifetime of intimate encounters with Mother Nature, both of which bring me seemingly endless sources of joy, discovery, and love.

NOTES

Introduction

1. Cambridge Dictionary. Definition of "disruptive" – English Dictionary. https://dictionary.cambridge.org/us/dictionary/english/disruptive. Accessed May 5, 2018.

2. Potter, Everett, quoting Shannon Stowell, from Five Myths About Adventure Travel. Special for USA Today. 2015. https://www.usatoday.com/story/travel/destinations/2015/08/24/adventure-travel/32131091/ Accessed May 5, 2018.

Part One: The Need for Creative Fitness Solutions

3. *Merck Manual,* pg 1643 – 1645

4. *Encyclopedia of Obesity and Eating Disorders.* Cassell, Dana, K., Larocca, Felix E.F., M.D., F.a.P.A. Facts on File. p. 139.

5. Hales CM, Carroll MD, Fryar CD, Ogden CL. Prevalence of obesity among adults and youth: United States, 2015-2016. NCHS data brief, no 288. Hyattsville, MD: National Center for Health Statistics, 2017. Pg 1. Retrieved from https://www.cdc.gov/nchs/data/databriefs/db288.pdf

6. National Center for Health Statistics. Health, United States, 2016; With Chartbook on Long-term Trends in Health. Hyattsville, MD. 2017. Pg 221. Retrieved from https://www.cdc.gov/nchs/data/hus/hus16.pdf#053

7. All definitions come from the *Diagnostic and Statistical Manual of Mental Disorders.* Fifth Edition. DSM-V. American Psychiatric Publishing.

8. Harvard Medical School, 2007. National Comorbidity Survey (NCS). Retrieved from https://www.hcp.med.harvard.edu/ncs/index.php. Data Table 2:12-month prevalence DSM-IV/WMH-CIDI disorders by sex and cohort. Accessed May 10, 2018.

9. Harvard Medical School, 2007. National Comorbidity Survey (NCS). Retrieved from https://www.hcp.med.harvard.edu/ncs/index.php. Data Table 1: Lifetime prevalence DSM-IV/WMH-CIDI disorders by sex and cohort. Accessed May 10, 2018.

10. Bloom, D.E. et al., 2011. The Global Economic Burden of Noncommunicable Diseases. Geneva: World Economic Forum. www3.weforum.org/docs/WEF_Harvard_HE/GlobalEconomicBurdenNoncommunicableDiseases_2011.pdf. Accessed May 10, 2018.

11. Pratt, L.A., Brody, D.J. Depression in the U.S. household population, 2009 – 2012. NCHS data brief, no 172. Hyattsville, MD: National Center for Health Statistics. 2014. Retrieved https://www.cdc.gov/nchs/data/databriefs/db172.pdf. Accessed May 10, 2018.

12. Archer, Shirley. 2013. Digital Distractions. IDEA Fitness Journal, Volume 10, Issue 6. Retrieved www.ideafit.com/fitness-library/digital-distractions. Accessed May 10, 2018.

13. Die With Me. Retrieved diewithme.online. Retrieved https://www.wsj.com/articles/your-phone-is-almost-out-of-battery-remain-calm-call-a-doctor-1525449283. Accessed May 10, 2018.

14 . Mickle, Tripp. May 4, 2018. Your Phone Is Almost Out of Battery. Remain Calm. Call A Doctor. Wall Street Journal.

15. Louv, Richard. Last Child in the Woods, Saving Our Children from Nature-Deficit Disorder. Algonquin Books of Chapel Hill. 2008. p. 36.

16. Robinson, Trip. April 12, 2013. *Faith, Religion, and the Environment.* Wallace Stegner Symposium. University of Utah.

17. Louv, Richard. Last Child in the Woods, Saving Our Children from Nature-Deficit Disorder. Algonquin Books of Chapel Hill. 2008. p. 367.

18. Miller, Elizabeth. Interior Sec. Sally Jewell outlines plan for engaging youth in outdoor industry. Snews. 2014. Retrieved from https://www.snewsnet.com/trade-

show/interior-sec-sally-jewell-outlines-plan-for-engagint-youth-in-outdoor-industry Accessed May 5, 2018.

19. Keeny, B.A. (Eds) (Aug. 2005) CBI Interview: Harvey Lauer, the man behind American Sports Data, Inc. Club Business International 24 (8), p. 42.

20. Rodriguez, Melissa. March 16, 2018. Latest Data Shows U.S. Health club Industry Serves 70.2 Million. The International Health, Racquet & sportsclub Association (IHRSA). Retrieved https://www.ihrsa.org/about/media-center/press-releases/latest-data-shows-u-s-health-club-industry-serves-70-2-million. Accessed May 12, 2018.

21. Physical Activity Council. 2018 Participation Report. Retrieved www.physicalactivitycouncil.com/pdfs/current.pdf. Accessed May 12, 2018.

Part Two: Mother Nature's Gym

22. Paine, Thomas. Major works: Common Sense / The American Crisis / The Rights of Man / The Age of Reason / Agrarian Justice. Lulu Press, Inc. 2017. p. 549.

23. Roberts, Michael. "The Touchy-Feely (But Totally Scientific!) Methods of Wallace. J. Nichols." *Outside Magazine*. December 2011.

24. Nichols, Wallace J. Blue Mind. The Surprising Science That Shows How Being On, In, near, or Under Water Can Make You Happier, Healthier, More Connected, and Better at What You Do. Little, Brown & Company. 2014

25. Nichols, Wallace J. Blue Mind. The Surprising Science That Shows How Being On, In, near, or Under Water Can Make You Happier, Healthier, More Connected, and Better at What You Do. Little, Brown & Company. 2014

26 . Williams, Florence. 2012. Take two hours of pine forest and call me in the morning. Outside Online. Retrieved from https://www.outsideonline.com/fitness/wellness/Take-Two-Hours-of-PineForest-and-Call-Me-in-the-Morning.html; accessed Jan. 10, 2013.

27. Williams, Florence. 2012. Take two hours of pine forest and call me in the morning. Outside Online. Retreived from https://www.outsideonline.com/fitness/wellness/Take-Two-Hours-of-PineForest-anc-Call-Me-in-the-Morning.html; accessed Jan. 10, 2013.

28. Abbey, Edward. The Journey Home: Some Words in Defense of the American West. New York, N.Y., U.S.A.: Plume, 1991. Print.

29. Edelin, William. A Spiritual Union, Mountain and Desert. The Desert Sun. 2011.

30. Johns Hopkins Medicine Health Library. Retrieved from http://www.hopkinsmedicine.org/healthlibrary/test_procedures/neurological/electro-encephalogram_eeg_92,P07655/

31. Yogananda, Paramahansa. Autobiography of a Yogi. Self Realization Fellowship. 1994. p. 265.

32. Zelaya, Rachel. What is the Meaning of OM? Retrieved from https://www.gaia.com/article/what-meaning-om; accessed May 13, 2018.

33. Die Hard Indian. Ancient rishis. Retrieved from diehardindian.com/ancient-rishis/. Accessed May 13, 2018.

34. Merejildo, James Arevalo. Inka Power Places. Solar Initiations. Mallku. 2007. p. 339.

35. Raytheon ITSS, et. Al. What is Schumann Resonance? Retrieved from http://image.gsfc.nasa.gov/poetry/ask/q768.html. Accessed May 13, 2018.

36. Garcia-Rill, Edgar, PhD. Waking and the Reticular Activating System in Health and Disease. Academic Press. 2012. Retrieved from https://www.sciencedirect.com/science/book/9780128013854#book-description. Accessed June 8, 2018.

37. Berry, Richard B., MD Fundamentals of Sleep Medicine. Saunders. 2012. Retrieved from https://www.sciencedirect.com/science/book/9781437703269#book-description. Accessed June 8, 2018.

38. Herrmann, Ned. What is the function of the various brainwaves? Scientific American. Retrieved from https://www.scientrificamerican/com/article/what-is-the-function-of-t-1997-12-22/ Accessed June 8, 2018.

39. Carson, Rachel. The Sense of Wonder. Harper & Row. 1956. p. 88.

40. Abrahamson, Jake. The Science of Awe. SIERRA Magazine. 2014.

41. Edelin, William. A Spiritual Union, Mountain and Desert. The Desert Sun. 2011. I received the newspaper clipping from a client in 2011. When I began the process of writing Mother Nature's Gym (then Sol Guide) in 2014 I reached out to Mr. Edelin in an email and we became pen pals. He sent me a number of his writings, including this one, which he wrote in August of 2011. Mr. Edelin died in 2015.

42. As I make my final edits to this course the short film Return from Desolation, created by Justin Clifton and Harlan Taney, is receiving rave reviews from spectators at environmental film festivals around the U.S. The movie is available online at https://www.desofilm.com and is a must-see for anyone interested in the topics of health and the outdoors and public lands.

Part Three: Sol Guide Method

43. Csikszentmihalyi, Mihaly. Flow The Psychology of Optimal Experience. New York: Harper & Row. 1990. p. 162.

44. Mumford, George. The Mindful Athlete: Secrets to Top Performance. Berkeley, California. Parallax Press. 2016. p. 71.

45 . Webb, Melanie. The Magic of Bali. ATHLETA chi blog. 2012. http://www.athleta.net/2012/03/05/the-magic-of-bali/

46. Brigham Young University Museum of Art. Gallery Guide. Exhibition Walk in Beauty. Hózho and Navajo Basketry. 2003.

47. Walk in Beauty: The Navajo and Their Blankets. Berlant, Anthony and Hunt Kahlenberg, Mary. New York Graphic Societ. Boston. 1977. Accessed http://booksoft-

hesouthwest.tumblr.com/post/21891165145/walk-in-beauty-the-navajo-and-their-blankets. Retrieved September, 2014.

Those reading this course as an e-book have a link to a recording by Jen Minkman-Saturay. I connected with Jen in 2014 as I wrote the first edition and found her song on YouTube. Print readers will find the link by visiting https://www.youtube.com/watch?v=vQG4qo1YHaE I personally don't sing and play guitar, but if I did this is one song I would learn to take on my outdoor fitness retreats to southern Utah!

48. World Health Organization, 2010. Global recommendations on physical activity for health. WHO Press, Geneva.

49. Louv, Richard. Last Child in the Woods: Saving Our Children from Nature-deficit Disorder. Chapel Hill, NC: Algonquin Books of Chapel Hill, 2008. p. 9.

50. Mate, Gabor. Scattered: How Attention Deficit Disorder Originates and What You Can Do About It. New York, New York: Plume, 2000. Print. p. 288.

51. Ludlow Christensen, Andrea. "Living the Playful Life." BYU Magazine 1 Aug. 2014. Print.

Part Four: The Outdoor Fitness Guide

52. Webb, Melanie. Slot Canyon Body Slam. CARSON Magazine. 2011.

53. Webb, Melanie. Mind, Body, and Spirit in Harmony. Athleta Chi Blog. Those reading this course as an e-book have a link to the complete article, while those reading the print edition can read it by visiting www.athleta.net/2012/11/08/mind-body-spirit-in-harmony

54. Webb, Melanie. Confessions of a Tour Guide. YourLifeIsATrip.com. 2014. If you're reading the e-book you have a link to take you to the complete article. Print readers can access the story by visiting https://www.yourlifeisatrip.com/home/confessions-of-a-tour-guide.html?rq+melanie%20webb

55. Louv, Richard. The Nature Principle: Human Restoration and the End of Nature-deficit Disorder. Chapel Hill, N.C.: Algonquin of Chapel Hill, 2011. Print.

Part Five: Creating Outdoor Fitness Retreats

56. Mother Nature's Gym. Webb, Melanie. *IDEA Fitness Journal.* May 2014. While I've cited my own article in this course, it's important to note that I did not invent the principle of FITT. Rather, it is a foundational principle outlined in personal training manuals.

57. Ratey, John, MD, SPARK, the Revolutionary New Science of Exercise and the Brain. Little, Brown and Company. 2008.

Part Six: Sol Guide Method Body-Weight Exercise Arsenal

For the sake of instruction and presentation I've grouped the exercises clusters and included them in the overall Sol Guide Method. However, as I'm sure most mind/body professionals and even lay people are aware, I certainly do not mean to imply that I invented or created the exercises presented. Unless cited otherwise in the chapter, the exercises selected are from the general body of exercises commonly used during a functional training or stretching workout.

PHOTO AND ILLUSTRATION CREDITS

Front and Back Cover Design & Illustration: Pascal Dangin
Back Cover Photo Inset: Pascal Dangin
How to Use this Book Photo: David Basset Photography
Part One Photo: David Basset Photography
Part Two Photo: Justin Clifton
Part Two Illustrations: Pete Iccabazzi
Part Three Photo: Earth River SUP featuring Greg 'Suggz' Miller and Cole Reintsma
   Part Three Photo: Jarred Ray Photography
Part Four Photo: Valerie Thompson Photography
Part Five Photo: Elizabeth Grey of Daybreak featuring Melanie Webb
Part Six Photo: Nina Larsen Reed featuring Amie Kane-Lee
  Sport photo collages: Sol Fitness Adventures trip highlights
  Exercise photo collages: Melanie Webb's exercise library
Part Six: Sol Guide Method Body-Weight Exercise Arsenal videos and editing:
  Brian Bunson, Videographer, Utah Media Services, and Aaron Gaitan, Director
  of Photography
About the Author: Victor Cooper Photography

ABOUT THE AUTHOR

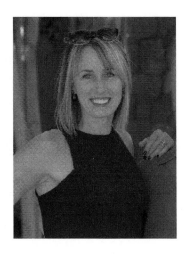

MELANIE WEBB is the Founder of Sol Fitness Adventures and luxury wellness retreat label WebbWell. She has spent her 20-year career working to help others live healthier, happier lives by sharing her knowledge and enthusiasm for fitness and outdoor adventure.

A Certified Personal Trainer through the American Council on Exercise (ACE), Melanie graduated with a B.S. in Physiology and Human Developmental Biology from Brigham Young University and took courses in Exercise Science, Nutrition, and Eating Behavior at The George Washington University. It was while pursuing her Master's Degree that Melanie began training clients at The Sports Club/LA in Washington, D.C. (now Equinox). She quickly realized that she didn't need another degree to do her best work, and she left academics to fully commit to her training practice. Before long Melanie's clients began to hire her to lead them on their own bucket list adventures. She drew upon her previous career experience and began to lead customized fitness retreats back to the remote landscapes she'd studied while working as a Wildlife Biologist for the State of Utah.

Melanie has compiled an impressive list of media appearances and contributions including *Denver Life, Fodor's, The Expert Vagabond, Adventure Sports Network, REAL SIMPLE, 805 Living, The Outsider by KUHL* and more. She has shared her expertise with tens of thousands of online readers as Assistant Editor of Exercise & Fitness at AllThingsHealing.com and as a presenter at the Women's Wellness Workshop at Canyon Ranch, Miami Beach (now Carillon Miami Wellness Resort).

An avid explorer, Melanie's work and personal athletic pursuits have taken her on active adventures around the globe. She remains committed to helping others challenge the body, lift the spirit, and engage the senses in wilderness at every opportunity. Melanie lives and works out of Salt Lake City, Utah.

Made in the USA
San Bernardino, CA
27 January 2020